HUNGER
FREE
FOREVER

HUNGER FREE FOREVER

THE NEW SCIENCE OF APPETITE CONTROL

**Michael T. Murray, N.D.,
and Michael R. Lyon, M.D.**

ATRIA BOOKS

NEW YORK   LONDON   TORONTO   SYDNEY

This publication contains the opinions and ideas of its authors. It is intended to provide helpful and informative material on the subjects addressed in the publication. It is sold with the understanding that the authors and publisher are not engaged in rendering medical, health, or any other kind of personal professional services in the book. The reader should consult his or her medical, health, or other competent professional before adopting any of the suggestions in this book or drawing inferences from it.

The authors and publisher specifically disclaim all responsibility for any liability, loss, or risk, personal or otherwise, which is incurred as a consequence, directly or indirectly, of the use and application of any of the contents of this book.

ATRIA BOOKS

A Division of Simon & Schuster, Inc.
1230 Avenue of the Americas
New York, NY 10020

Copyright © 2007 by Michael T. Murray, n.d., and Michael Lyon, M.D.

All rights reserved, including the right to reproduce this book
or portions thereof in any form whatsoever.
For information address Atria Books Subsidiary Rights Department,
1230 Avenue of the Americas, New York, NY 10020.

First Atria Books hardcover edition December 2007

ATRIA BOOKS and colophon are trademarks of Simon & Schuster, Inc.

For information about special discounts for bulk purchases,
please contact Simon & Schuster Special Sales at
1-800-456-6798 or business@simonandschuster.com.

Recipes appearing in Chapter 11 are reprinted courtesy of www.recipezaar.com.

Designed by Karolina Harris

Manufactured in the United States of America

10   9   8   7   6   5   4   3   2   1

Library of Congress Cataloging-in-Publication Data
Murray, Michael T.
    Hunger free forever : the new science of appetite control / Michael T. Murray and Michael R. Lyon.
        p.   cm.
    Includes index.
    1. Reducing diets. 2. Reducing diets–Recipes. 3. Weight loss. 4. Appetite. I. Lyon, Michael R. II. Title.
    RM222.2.M846 2007
    613.2'5–dc22   2007034140

ISBN-13: 978-1-4165-4904-8
ISBN-10:   1-4165-4904-8

To everyone who has ever
sincerely tried to lose weight and failed

CONTENTS

HUNGER
FREE
FOREVER

INTRODUCTION:

THE PROMISE OF HIGH SATIETY

You are about to discover that the key to effective and lasting weight loss is not dieting or deprivation, but rather eliminating excessive hunger and increasing the feelings of pleasure and satisfaction from food. The Hunger Free Forever program provides a near effortless program for safe, effective, and lifelong weight control that has evolved from major scientific discoveries we have made in the field of appetite regulation. Our discoveries have been effectively applied in community weight-loss programs conducted over the past few years on hundreds of people. This simple approach allows you to reach and easily maintain your body weight goals utilizing exciting new scientific breakthroughs to normalize your appetite and consistently enjoy a high degree of satiety from the food you eat.

Satiety is defined as the state of being full or gratified to the point of satisfaction. Research has shown that humans eat to achieve satiety and those who are overweight have an increased frequency of food cravings and a resistance to satiety after eating adequate amounts of food. Our program uncovers the reasons for this resistance to satiety and increased food craving and provides the vital keys to restoring normal appetite control—whether you want to lose 5 pounds or 200 pounds.

If you have struggled to achieve your ideal body weight, if you have tried various diets only to end up weighing more than when you started, if you feel that if you simply look at food that it magically winds up on your thighs, or if you always feel like you are hungry and never satisfied, the Hunger Free Forever program is for you.

BOB'S STORY

For the first time in my life I have hope and confidence that I can reach my desired weight. I still have a long way to go, but I have lost 45 pounds in the last three months following your program. What is so amazing to me is that I have been battling my weight my whole life and have tried every diet imaginable, yet this is the first time I have ever really known what it feels like to be satisfied and not hungry. It is just an amazing feeling for me. While I could follow a diet perfectly during the day, once I started eating at dinner it seemed that I could not stop until I went to sleep. Now, that switch has definitely turned off. Thank you is simply not enough to express my deep appreciation.

Bob, age 45

This program is truly different than any other. Unlike all of the popular diets, we reveal specific eating strategies and appetite-reducing discoveries that eliminate unhealthy food cravings and create a high level of satiety even with significant reductions in caloric intake. Just think about it: If you feel satisfied, eating fewer calories is not deprivation. In fact, followers of our program gain an even greater appreciation and love for food. By retraining appetite and metabolism, you can change your relationship with food from unhealthy and excessive to healthy and moderate. It is a liberating experience.

THE HUNGER FREE FOREVER PROGRAM GOALS AND PRINCIPLES

We have discovered one of the keys to long-term weight-loss success is learning how to live a better life through enjoying better nutrition. The success is found by consuming special foods, fiber combinations, and dietary supplements designed to promote satiety and burn fat (thermogenesis). The beauty of the Hunger Free Forever program is that it is simple, easy to follow, and highly effective. It promotes weight loss because it is based upon achieving several important goals:

- Decreasing appetite and calories consumed.
- Normalizing and stabilizing blood glucose levels.
- Increasing metabolism and the burning of fat, while preserving muscle mass—all without the use of hazardous stimulants.
- Resetting the mechanisms that control individual fat cell size and body weight.
- Adjusting food and lifestyle choices to promote ideal body weight and create a healthier relationship with food.

Specifically, you learn how to:

- Utilize a newly discovered, commercially available blend of highly viscous soluble fiber known as PolyGlycopleX (PGX) with or before each meal to improve blood sugar control.
- Take advantage of foods and recipes that promote satiety and reduce caloric intake.
- Enjoy foods that promote lean body mass, improve blood sugar control, provide the right type of fats, and reduce inflammation.
- Regularly consume special foods that increase metabolism, reduce appetite, and improve insulin action.
- Utilize appropriate natural products to assist with weight loss. You will learn to evaluate your need for and use of products that promote thermogenesis, lower elevated cortisol and reduce stress-induced eating, increase insulin sensitivity and improve blood sugar control, and reduce appetite.
- Build lean muscle mass through exercise, diet, and nutritional supplementation.
- Program and condition the mind to achieve success.

A SCIENTIFIC APPROACH

The Hunger Free Forever program features principles and components that have been well studied and proven effective through years of clinical research and community weight-loss programs. It applies the most salient principles from scientific evaluations on diet and weight loss to eliminate the tremendous confusion our society has about eating. Most of all, it applies these principles in a simple, practical, and no-nonsense fashion for people whose lives are too busy to be governed by rigid diets. While it is true that most popular diets promote short-term weight loss if followed closely, the majority of people fail to achieve and maintain their weight-loss goals. Why? Other diets focus on rigid and usually impractical dietary schemes that do little or nothing to eliminate unhealthy food cravings and excessive hunger.

Instead, this program represents the new frontier of achieving and maintaining weight loss. Its effects occur at every major level of appetite control. In particular, it focuses on improving blood sugar control. Mounting research points to the important role that blood sugar plays in the regulation of human appetite. Much of the effect of blood sugar fluctuations on appetite control can be traced to specialized immune cells, called glial cells, that surround every brain cell. Glial cells are important in sensing the level of glucose in the blood. Every time blood sugar drops rapidly in a short span of time, glial cells send powerful signals to brain regions such as the hypothalamus, which are interpreted as a desire to initiate food intake. Because of insulin resistance and its accompanying poor glucose regulation, overweight people spend their days riding a virtual blood sugar roller coaster. As a result, they experience potentially hundreds of neurological commands to eat, most of which are inappropriate. The Hunger Free Forever program gets people off the blood sugar roller coaster within a few days; the frequency and magnitude of these intense desires to eat are greatly diminished or eliminated all together. Thus satiety can then be achieved and maintained, leading to safe and effective weight loss.

By using new techniques in twenty-four-hour blood sugar monitoring, our research has, for the first time, documented that excessive appetite and food cravings in overweight subjects are directly correlated with rapid fluctuations in blood glucose throughout the day and night. Furthermore, we have documented that our program dramatically restores the body's ability to control blood sugar levels and that this accomplishment is powerfully linked to remarkable improvements in insulin sensitivity and reductions in appetite.

SARAH'S STORY

For the past seven years my life was a living hell. Each day I awakened feeling terrible and with the resolve that I would finally "get it together," but it just never seemed to happen. After my car accident, I was unable to exercise and I gained 40 pounds in just over four months. Once I hit 200 pounds, my appetite seemed out of control. I had complete control through the day, skipping breakfast and eating mostly salad for lunch, but after dinner everything changed and I seemed to have insatiable cravings for food, especially things that were very salty or very sweet. On top of that, every night I would awaken at 2:00 to 3:00 a.m. with a horrible gnawing feeling in my stomach and an urgent need to eat, which I began to do, and did, almost every night since. Nothing helped me. Dieting made things much worse and I have never been able to endure diets for more than a few days. I was so ashamed of this behavior that I hid it from my family and suffered alone. That is, until you heard my story and seemed to think that this was a common problem and one that could be helped. When you showed me my blood sugar graph, I was amazed at how up-and-down it was, especially how fast my blood sugar dropped in the middle of the night. You relieved so much guilt when I understood that my problem was physical and very real.

I am happy to report that within three days of starting the Hunger Free Forever program, I slept through the night for the first time in years and have done so since. I now awaken energized and hungry for breakfast in the morning and I don't have any sweet tooth at all! I get comfortably hungry by meal times, but rarely ever have cravings between meals like I used to. Since I was almost 300 pounds, I know I have a long road ahead, but this program is so comfortable that I feel like I can eat like this for the rest of my life even though I am losing so much weight that people don't recognize me now. I will always be grateful for your help and your wisdom.

Sarah, age 48

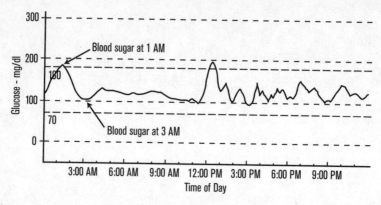

Figure 1. Sarah's 24-hour blood sugar graph before the Hunger Free Forever program.

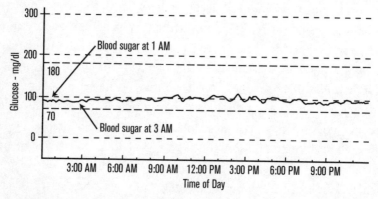

Figure 2. Sarah's 24-hour blood sugar graph 4 weeks after starting the Hunger Free Forever Program.

The principal reason why the Hunger Free Forever program brings about a remarkable normalization in blood sugar control is that it restores insulin sensitivity better than any drug or dietary program ever studied. With restored insulin sensitivity, appetite is controlled—leading to healthier food choices—and metabolism is increased, promoting fat loss and muscle growth.

PGX–THE SUPERSOLUBLE FIBER

The key aid to losing weight safely, effectively, and permanently is to greatly increase the consumption of dietary fiber. Unfortunately, to achieve the full appetite stabilizing effects of fiber, very large quantities of fiber must be consumed—higher quantities than most people would ever eat. Most North Americans consume 5 to 15 grams of fiber per day. The United States Department of Agriculture (USDA) recommends at least 30 grams per day. In reality, 50 to 75 grams or more of conventional dietary fiber per day would likely be required in order to have highly significant effects on satiety in overweight individuals.

The effectiveness of fiber on reducing appetite, blood sugar, and cholesterol is directly proportionate to the amount of water the fiber is able to absorb (water-holding capacity) and the degree of thickness or viscosity it imparts when in the stomach and intestine. For instance, this solubility is why oat bran lowers cholesterol and controls blood sugar better, gram for gram, than wheat bran. With this in mind, researchers have been seeking to identify and isolate dietary fibers with the highest viscosity and water-holding capacity in order to make them available as food ingredients or nutritional supplements. What they have found is that certain fibers, when combined, actually synergize and multiply each other's effects. Thus, specific fiber combinations, gram for gram, may exert health effects equivalent to larger gram quantities of similar fibers when consumed alone.

Although there are many varieties of soluble fiber, a completely novel blend known as PolyGlycopleX (PGX) is the most viscous and soluble fiber ever discovered. The fibers in PGX work synergistically to produce a higher level of viscosity, gel-forming properties, and expansion with water than with the same quantity of any other fiber alone. The blend is able to bind roughly hundreds of times its weight in water, resulting in a volume and viscosity three to five times greater than other highly soluble fibers like psyllium or oat beta glucan. To put this in perspective: A small 5-gram serving of PGX in a meal replacement formula or on its own produces a volume and viscosity that would be equal to as much as four bowls of oat bran. In this way, small quantities of PGX can be added to foods or taken as a drink before meals to have an impact on appetite and blood sugar control equivalent to eating enormous and impractical quantities of any other form of fiber.

The development of PGX is the result of intense scientific research at the University of Toronto led by Dr. David Jenkins, Dr. Tom Wolever,

Dr. Alexandra Jenkins, and Dr. Vladimir Vuksan, discoverers of the now-popular glycemic index. This world-recognized research team tested hundreds of different fiber combinations in laboratory, animal, and human studies before the basic composition of this super fiber was discovered. Coauthor Dr. Michael Lyon, director of the Canadian Center for Functional Medicine, and the team of nutritional scientists at Natural Factors then conducted two years of exhaustive research to create the processes and formulas that led to the patent-pending ingredient PGX. Dr. Lyon continues to collaborate with the University of Toronto on PGX research. In fact, recent studies have shown that when added to virtually any food with a high glycemic index, PGX can reduce the glycemic index of the food by an amazing 50 to 70 percent.

Detailed clinical studies published in major medical journals and presented at the world's major diabetes conferences have shown PGX to:

- Reduce appetite and promote effective weight loss, even in the morbidly obese.
- Increase the level of compounds that block the appetite and promote satiety.
- Decrease the level of compounds that stimulate overeating.
- Reduce postprandial (after-meal) blood glucose levels when added to or taken with foods.
- Reduce the glycemic index of any food or beverage.
- Increase insulin sensitivity and decrease blood insulin levels better than any drug.
- Improve diabetes control and dramatically reduce the need for medications or insulin in the diabetic.
- Stabilize blood sugar control in the overweight and obese.
- Lower blood cholesterol and triglycerides.

DR. MURRAY AS A GUINEA PIG

For nearly twenty years my body weight fluctuated from between 200 and 208 pounds. I am 6'1" tall and fairly muscular, so I carried that weight well. But I decided that prior to the pilot study Dr. Lyon was

ANTHONY'S STORY

I'd like to take this opportunity to thank you and your staff for introducing me to PGX. For many years I tried a variety of products on the market to aid my constant battle with weight and have always been let down. After being on PGX for only five months, I've lost 37 pounds, regained my livelihood, and have gained my life back.

It feels great to know that my cholesterol level is back to normal, not to mention that I've gone from a size 44 waist to a size 34. All of my customers and fellow employees have seen me go from 254 pounds to 217 pounds and want to know what my secret is. I've told them it's not a secret: it's about believing in yourself and getting a little help from PGX. Plus, I have a personal goal to get back to less than 200 pounds within a year and I know I can achieve this now.

Using PGX on a daily basis—twice a day for me—is so easy. I use it like a salt replacement on my meals, which are well balanced. I can also exercise regularly again, and I feel great. Again, thank you, I am living proof that with PGX, if you want to lose weight you can do it.

Anthony, age 38

conducting at the Canadian Center for Functional Medicine featuring some of the key principles and components of our program, I would serve as a human guinea pig to see if the program would be easy to follow, and what sort of results participants might expect.

I am glad I did, because it was a life-changing experience. On August 18, 2003, I weighed 206 pounds with a body fat percentage of 21.3. Four weeks later, I weighed in at 188—my lowest weight in fifteen years! Now, I would normally tell people that amount of weight loss is not wise because it usually is associated with a loss of muscle mass, but because my scale also determines body fat percentage, I learned that my body fat decreased from 22.3 percent to 17.8 percent. So most of the weight loss was actually fat loss. As incredible as it was to lose so much weight so rapidly (even though I had only planned on getting down to 195 pounds), what was really amazing to me was that the whole process was *effortless*. I felt satisfied all the time because I was using PGX to reduce my appetite. In the four years since going on the program, my weight has stabilized between 188 and 190 pounds, and—amazingly—my body fat percentage now fluctuates between 8 and 10 percent. To put this into perspective, I have lost over 28 pounds of fat while actually adding over 10 pounds of muscle. So, I know firsthand that following the program given in *Hunger Free Forever* not only helps people lose the weight, but continuing to follow the principles allows them to keep it off and even continue to burn more fat and build more lean muscle mass, a key goal for long-term health and vitality.

GETTING STARTED

Our experience is that most people lose up to four pounds the first week. After this initial weight loss, they usually lose between one and two and a half pounds per week. More weight loss is possible on this program, but we simply do not recommend it. Severe caloric restriction is quite easy when following the guidelines of our program, but when you lose weight too rapidly it means a lot of muscle mass loss as well. Since muscle mass is very important in long-term health, it is critical that it be maintained, or better yet actually increased. Gradual weight loss, combined with exercise to build muscle mass, is the ideal, long-term solution to weight management.

To help motivate you to begin, keep this checklist of benefits of the Hunger Free Forever program handy. The program works because it:

- Corrects the body's attempt to hold onto fat in response to reduced calorie intake.
- Focuses on eating strategies, specific foods, and dietary supplements that improve blood sugar control and increase the natural release of satiety-inducing hormones.
- Utilizes measures effectively to increase the burning of fat and preserve metabolic rate even when cutting calories.
- Increases lean body mass (muscle) while burning large amounts of fat.

- Can be easily followed and adhered to as a permanent and pleasurable way of life.
- Provides clear direction, recipes, menu plans, and methods to keep to the program when traveling or eating out.

Are you ready to let the Hunger Free Forever program work for you? Now is a good time to reveal the healthy person inside of you.

1

WHY IS THE WORLD
GROWING FAT?

Throughout history, malnutrition, hunger, and even famine have been unwelcome yet frequent companions of humankind. Over the past fifty years, unrivaled changes in food technology, transportation, and agriculture have created an unprecedented increase in the availability of food throughout the world. Because of this, obesity now outranks malnutrition even in most developing countries. According to the World Health Organization (WHO), out of the world's six billion people, one billion are overweight, compared to 800 million who are undernourished. Even Africa, a continent usually synonymous with hunger, is falling prey to obesity. More than 33.3 percent of African women and 25 percent of African men are estimated to be overweight, and the WHO predicts that these numbers will rise to 41 percent and 30 percent respectively in the next ten years.

In the developed world, obesity is a true epidemic. North America has the highest percentage of people who are obese, as well as the highest number of people who are succumbing to obesity-related illnesses. Our healthcare system is already strained by this epidemic, and the ability to sustain even basic healthcare in the years to come is in doubt if obesity continues to prevail as it does today. We all need to do our part in helping to reverse this worrisome trend. The best place to start is in our own homes and our own lives. Helping to face weight problems head-on and giving the tools to solve them is what this book is all about.

OBESITY DEFINED

The simplest definition of obesity is an excessive amount of body fat. Obesity is not the same as being overweight, which refers to an excess of body weight relative to height. For example, a muscular athlete may be overweight, yet have a low body-fat percentage. With this distinction in mind, it is obvious that using body weight alone as an index of obesity is not entirely accurate. Nonetheless, a simple measure known as the body mass index (BMI) is now the accepted standard for classifying individuals with regard to their body composition. BMI generally correlates well to a person's total body fat. The BMI is calculated by dividing a person's weight in kilograms by height squared in meters. The mathematical formula is "kg/m^2." Now, we know that you are not likely to calculate your BMI, so here is a simple table to use. Find your height in the left-hand column. Move across the row to the your weight. The number at the top of that column is the BMI for your height and weight.

A BMI between 25 and 29.9 is a marker for being overweight, while obesity is defined as a BMI of 30 or greater. A BMI of 40 or greater is referred to as morbid obesity and is associated with extreme health risks. To put the BMI in perspective: A 5'4" woman with a BMI of 30 is about 30 pounds above her ideal body weight. So, obesity is not a matter of simply being a few pounds overweight. It reflects a significant amount of excess fat.

There is one more calculation that is important for determining overall health: your waist size. The combination of your BMI and your waist circumference is a very good indicator of your risk for all of the diseases associated with obesity, especially the major killers like heart disease, strokes, cancer, and diabetes.

BODY FAT VERSUS BODY WEIGHT

The number on your scale represents your total weight, not the relationship of fat to muscle or body composition. While being overweight is a risk factor for type 2 diabetes, it is not the critical risk factor. Correctly stated, it is increased body fat that is associated with type 2 dia-

BODY MASS INDEX (BMI) CHART

BMI (kg/m²)	19	20	21	22	23	24	25	26	27	28	29	30	35	40
Height (in.)	Weight (lb.)													
58	91	96	100	105	110	115	119	124	129	134	138	143	167	191
59	94	99	104	109	114	119	124	128	133	138	143	148	173	198
60	97	102	107	112	118	123	128	133	138	143	148	153	179	204
61	100	106	111	116	122	127	132	137	143	148	153	158	185	211
62	104	109	115	120	126	131	136	142	147	153	158	164	191	218
63	107	113	118	124	130	135	141	146	152	158	163	169	197	225
64	110	116	122	128	134	140	145	151	157	163	169	174	204	232
65	114	120	126	132	138	144	150	156	162	168	174	180	210	240
66	118	124	130	136	142	148	155	161	167	173	179	186	216	247
67	121	127	134	140	146	153	159	166	172	178	185	191	223	255
68	125	131	138	144	151	158	164	171	177	184	190	197	230	262
69	128	135	142	149	155	162	169	176	182	189	196	203	236	270
70	132	139	146	153	160	167	174	181	188	195	202	207	243	278
71	136	143	150	157	165	172	179	186	193	200	208	215	250	286
72	140	147	154	162	169	177	184	191	199	206	213	221	258	294
73	144	151	159	166	174	182	189	197	204	212	219	227	265	302
74	148	155	163	171	179	186	194	202	210	218	225	233	272	311
75	152	160	168	176	184	192	200	208	216	224	232	240	279	319
76	156	164	172	180	189	197	205	213	221	230	238	246	287	328

betes, not increased body weight. While there is a strong correlation between body weight and body fat content, people of normal body weight can develop type 2 diabetes if they have an increased body fat percentage, especially if that excess fat is collecting around the waist or gut. That spare tire accumulation of fat can lead to what is referred to as "metabolic obesity."

To determine body composition more accurately, we recommend using a scale that utilizes a safe, low level amount of electricity, known as bioelectrical impedance, to determine body fat percentage. Since fat

RISK OF ASSOCIATED DISEASE ACCORDING TO BMI AND WAIST SIZE

BMI	Classification	Waist less than or equal to 40 in. (men) or 35 in. (women)	Waist greater than 40 in. (men) or 35 in. (women)
18.5 or less	Underweight	—	N/A
18.5–24.9	Normal	—	N/A
25.0–29.9	Overweight	Increased	High
30.0–34.9	Obese	High	Very High
35.0–39.9	Obese	Very High	Very High
40 or greater	Extremely Obese	Extremely High	Extremely High

does not conduct much bioelectricity, a higher degree of impedance of the electrical charge is associated with higher body fat percentage. The most popular scales of this sort are manufactured by Tanita (www. tanita.com) and range in cost from $55 to $200 depending upon desired features. Another, less expensive option is the Accu-Measure skin caliper. This is a simple tool that lets you estimate your body fat percentage by measuring the fat under the skin of the abdomen (www.ac cumeasurefitness.com). Ideally, women should strive to keep their body fat percentage below 25 percent and men below 20 percent.

Obesity Is the Biggest Threat to America

In 1962, the percentage of obesity in America's population was at 13 percent. By 1980 it had risen to 15 percent, by 1994 to 23 percent, and by the year 2004 the obesity progression in America had reached a rate of one out of three or 33 percent. Approximately 65 million adult Americans are now obese—more than the total populations of Britain, France, or Italy. As alarming as these statistics are, it must be pointed out that there is no end in sight. This trend is still rising rapidly. In particular, the percentage of children who are obese is rising at an alarming rate.

While terrorism, environmental pollution, and dwindling natural resources certainly put the future of our nation in peril, a very strong case can be made for the obesity epidemic being ranked as the most

BODY FAT RATING CHART FOR USE
WITH A BODY FAT MEASURING SCALE

Male

Age	Risky	Excellent	Good	Fair	Poor
19–24	<6%	10.8%	14.9%	19.0%	23.3%
25–29	<6%	12.8%	16.5%	20.3%	24.4%
30–34	<6%	14.5%	18.0%	21.5%	25.2%
35–39	<6%	16.1%	19.4%	22.6%	26.1%
40–44	<6%	17.5%	20.5%	23.6%	26.9%
45–49	<6%	18.6%	21.5%	24.5%	27.6%
50–54	<6%	19.8%	22.7%	25.6%	28.7%
55–59	<6%	20.2%	23.2%	26.2%	29.3%
60+	<6%	20.3%	23.5%	26.7%	29.8%

Female

Age	Risky	Excellent	Good	Fair	Poor
19–24	<9%	18.9%	22.1%	25.0%	29.6%
25–29	<9%	18.9%	22.0%	25.4%	29.8%
30–34	<9%	19.7%	22.7%	26.4%	30.5%
35–39	<9%	21.0%	24.0%	27.7%	31.5%
40–44	<9%	22.6%	25.6%	29.3%	32.8%
45–49	<9%	24.3%	27.3%	30.9%	34.1%
50–54	<9%	26.6%	29.7%	33.1%	36.2%
55–59	<9%	27.4%	30.7%	34.0%	37.3%
60+	<9%	27.6%	31.0%	34.4%	38.0%

significant threat to the future of the United States as well as other nations. Obesity is now regarded as the major cause of death in the United States. This epidemic has been fueled by many factors, including the collusion between the food industry and the U.S. government. Without question, American baby boomers and the generations that have followed have been led to the trough of obesity and told to indulge with pleasure by the food industry as well as the policies of the U.S. government. Food companies and the fast-food industry have used marketing as well as the science of food technology to trigger wanton gluttony in a way that is eerily similar to the methods the tobacco companies employed to develop more addictive cigarettes. The food industry, through lobbying, coercion, greed, and advertising, has influenced us to make dietary choices that fatten us up and harm our health.

HEALTH RISKS ASSOCIATED WITH OBESITY

CARDIOVASCULAR SYSTEM
- Chronic venous insufficiency, varicose veins
- Hypertension
- Hyperlipidemia (high cholesterol and triglycerides)
- Atherosclerosis
- Deep vein thrombosis
- Peripheral vascular disease

DIGESTIVE SYSTEM
- Gastroesophageal reflux disease (heartburn)
- Gallbladder disease
- Nonalcoholic steatohepatitis (fatty liver disease)

ENDOCRINE SYSTEM
- Type 2 diabetes
- Pancreatitis

MUSCULOSKELETAL SYSTEM
- Osteoarthritis
- Rheumatoid arthritis
- Vertebral disk herniation
- Degenerative joint disease
- Inguinal hernia
- Low back pain

NERVOUS SYSTEM
- Carpal tunnel syndrome
- Stroke
- Dementia
- Depression

REPRODUCTIVE SYSTEM
- Infertility
- Menstrual abnormalities
- Pregnancy abnormalities
- Hirsutism (female masculinization)
- Impotence
- Polycystic ovary syndrome (PCOS)
- Neural tube birth defects
- Infertility

RESPIRATORY SYSTEM
- Asthma
- Obesity hypoventilation syndrome
- Sleep apnea
- Pulmonary hypertension

URINARY SYSTEM
- Urinary stress incontinence
- Increased uric acid
- Renal disease

DERMATOLOGIC SYSTEM (SKIN)	IMMUNE SYSTEM
• Cellulitis (inflammation or infection of the connective tissue of the skin) • Fungal skin infections	• Cancers (breast, prostate, and colon) • Poor healing of wounds and infection

THE EXPORTATION OF OBESITY

So what is the biggest contributor to the rising obesity rates world-wide? Without a doubt it is the rise in popularity of American food—and not just fast food, but also soft drinks like Coke and Pepsi, and other food and beverages laden with high fructose corn syrup (HFCS). In fact, many experts believe that the large increase in the use of HFCS in the past thirty years is directly related to the overall increase in sugar consumption in the United States. It is also being linked to both the obesity and diabetes epidemics. This link was detailed exceptionally well in *Fat Land: How Americans Became the Fattest People in the World* by Greg Critser.

With a quick search on the Internet you will find HFCS referred to as "the Devil's candy," a "sinister invention," and "the crack of sweeteners." A distant derivative of corn, the highly processed syrup was created in the late 1960s and has become a hard-to-avoid staple of the American diet over the last twenty-five years.

Many different products use HFCS as an ingredient. It provides the sweetness in everything from soft drinks like 7Up and root beer; fruit beverages like Snapple; and most baked goods including cookies, crackers, bread, and even ketchup. Food companies use large quantities of HFCS because it is very cheap. A single 12-ounce can of Coke or Pepsi has as much as 13 teaspoons of sugar in the form of HFCS. And because the amount of soda we drink has more than doubled since 1970 to about 56 gallons per person a year, so has the amount of HFCS we consume. In 2001, we ate or drank almost 63 pounds of it, according to the USDA. That translates to an average of 31 teaspoons a day, and at 16 calories per teaspoon represents a daily intake of 496 calories. Most Americans consume 45 percent of their daily calories in the form of sugar and HFCS. This dietary pattern is at the center of the storm of obesity sweeping the United States and other countries around the world.

The bottom line is that obesity is principally caused by eating more calories than are utilized by the body. Too many of America's food choices are high in calories, but low on satiety—chief among these culprits are soft drinks and other sources of HFCS. As a result, the infiltration of the American diet, beverages, and lifestyle into other parts of the world is creating a potential worldwide catastrophic effect on

FOOD FACT: EVEN DIET DRINKS PROMOTE OBESITY

In a landmark analysis, Dr. Matthias B. Schulze of the Harvard School of Public Health and colleagues examined the relationships between sugar-sweetened beverage consumption and weight gain and diabetes risk in women. What they found was not surprising. Weight gain was highest among women who increased their sugar-sweetened soft drink consumption from one or fewer drinks per week to one or more drinks per day. This change resulted in an average weight gain of nearly 2½ pounds per year or about 10 pounds over a four-year period. In addition, women consuming one or more sugar-sweetened soft drinks per day had an 83-percent increased risk for type 2 diabetes compared with those who consumed less than one of these beverages per month.

So you might think that the answer is to switch to diet sodas, right? Unfortunately, it's not that simple. Research at the University of Texas actually showed that in an eight-year study, 55 percent of those subjects who drank 12 to 24 ounces of diet sodas daily became overweight—about twice as many as those consuming regular soft drinks with HFCS. In other words, diet soda consumption is twice as likely to lead to obesity as consuming soft drinks sweetened with HFCS. Why? Because it appears the diet drinks confuse the appetite control centers to trigger hunger rather than promote satiety.

health with dramatically increased rates of obesity, type 2 diabetes, and virtually ever other chronic disease.

IS OBESITY INHERITED?

Yes and no. While there is no actual "fat gene," virtually all of us have inherited a powerful tendency toward obesity. It actually begins at the moment of conception as the genetic code from our parents combine. This tendency is mostly in the form of survival mechanisms built into our normal physiology. And, although there may or may not be a specific fat gene, the tendency to be overweight is definitely magnified by the presence of obesity in our parents. If one of our parents was obese, we have an uphill battle in life with obesity. If both parents were obese, it is an uphill battle with a fifty-pound backpack—a little harder, but not impossible. Like most health conditions, however, while there may be a genetic tendency toward obesity or thinness, environmental and dietary factors are more important. For an example, let's take a look at the case of the Pima Indians.

A century ago, the Pima Indians, native to Arizona, were a lean and wiry people. Obesity was unknown to them. In fact, they had no word in their vocabulary to describe being fat. Once placed on reservations, they were no longer faced with periodic food shortages. As the Bureau of Indian Affairs provided them with flour, sugar, oil, and corn, an astonishing thing happened. These lean and wiry people developed an astronomical incidence of obesity. At one time, 100 percent of adult Pima Indians were grossly obese and the incidence of type 2 diabetes was a staggering 65 percent. The numbers have come down a bit (70 percent and 22 percent, respectively), but are still among the highest in the world.

In 1962, anthropologist James V. Neel suggested that tribal hunter-gathers like the Pimas had body processes well adapted to feast-or-famine cycles. This genetic adaptation was termed the "thrifty genotype" to signify the ability to withstand famines. During periods of famine, those of Pima forebearers whose bodies were not thrifty or capable of storing enough energy to survive without food died out. Those who survived were those who could survive long periods without food.

They possessed a thrifty genotype and subsequently continued to pass this genetic tendency to their children.

To illustrate just how powerful the thrifty gene can be in helping to survive a famine, let's look to some studies done in the early 1950s in a strain of chronically obese mice. When these mice were allowed an unlimited food supply, they would balloon and add as much as half the body weight of normal mice. When these fat mice were deprived of food they survived an average of forty days while normal mice would only live for ten days at the most.

The basic underlying mechanism in the chronically obese mice and Pima Indians with the thrifty gene is a natural craving for carbohydrates that causes consumption of them whenever they are available, even if hunger is not present. They also possessed the ability to make more insulin and store the excess calories consumed as fat. Pima Indians with the thrifty genotype also easily develop resistance to insulin when they consume excess carbohydrates. What this additional mechanism produces is an even greater ability to store fat and as a result enables them to live through famines. With time, the survival of the fittest led to virtually an entire culture possessing the thrifty gene.

Throughout the history of the world the ability to express the thrifty genotype was rewarded with survival. As a result, this genetic predisposition is one of the critical factors fueling the obesity epidemic.

PHENOTYPE VERSUS GENOTYPE

Even with the presence of the thrifty genotype, diet and lifestyle are the critical factors in determining obesity and diabetes. To illustrate this fact, all that we have to do is compare the rate of diabetes and obesity of Pima Indians living in Arizona to those living in isolated regions of Mexico who still cultivate corn, beans, and potatoes as their main staples, plus a limited amount of seasonal vegetables and fruits such as zucchini, squash, tomatoes, garlic, green peppers, peaches, and apples. The Pimas of Mexico also make heavy use of wild and medicinal plants in their diet. They work hard, have no electricity or running water in their homes, and walk long distances to bring in drinking water or to wash their clothes. They use no modern household devices; consequently, food preparation and household chores require extra effort by the women. In contrast, the Pima Indians of Arizona are largely sedentary and follow the dietary practices of typical Americans.

The differences are astounding. Even when the obesity and type 2 diabetes rates of adult Arizona Pimas were at an all-time high of 100 percent and 65 percent, respectively, the rates in the Mexican Pimas were significantly lower—obesity was less than 10 percent and type 2 diabetes was virtually nonexistent.

Remarkably, the Mexican Pimas are able to avoid obesity even when consuming a diet rich in carbohydrates. The secret to their diet is not that it is high in carbohydrates, but that it consists of whole, unprocessed foods, loaded with fiber. In fact, the Mexican Pimas have been enjoying the benefits of a high satiety diet, a diet that keeps them feeling full without overfilling them with calories.

Further evidence that diet and lifestyle appear to be able to overcome even the strongest genetic predisposition is some of the intervention studies with Pima Indians. When placed on a more traditional diet along with physical exercise, blood sugar levels improve dramatically and weight loss occurs. The focus right now by various medical organizations such as the National Institutes of Health to combat the epidemic of diabetes and obesity in the Pima Indians is to educate children on the importance of exercise and dietary choices to reduce the risk of type 2 diabetes.

The reason why diet and lifestyle are so much more important than genetic factors in influencing body weight, insulin sensitivity, and type 2 diabetes is the difference between the genotype and its actual expression, phenotype. Genotype refers to a particular genetic code. Phenotype, on the other hand, represents the actual expression of the genetic information. For example, even though identical twins have the exact same genetic information, they have different fingerprints.

With the thrifty genotype, there is an even higher degree of "phenotypic plasticity." What this term signifies is the relative expression of the genotype. If the genotype is always expressed no matter what the environmental or dietary factors are, then it would have little phenotypic plasticity. On the other hand, if the expression of the genotype is greatly influenced by environmental or dietary factors, then it would have a very high degree of phenotypic plasticity. While virtually all of us now have genotypes or genetic codes that set us for obesity, the reality is that if we take appropriate dietary and lifestyle steps we can block the expression of the thrifty genotype that can lead to obesity and type 2 diabetes.

DR. LYON'S LESSONS LEARNED FROM WORKING IN NATIVE COMMUNITIES

Back in the mid 1980s I had a chance to gain some firsthand experience working with Native Americans as a resident physician at one of the largest "Indian" hospitals in the U.S. Public Health System in Oklahoma. Over the three years of my residency, I spent many months and uncountable 100-plus-hour workweeks serving the people of the surrounding Native communities. As a struggling resident, I could not justify the expense of driving my car thirty-five miles each day to work, and so I rode my bicycle back and forth along the hot and hilly roads of eastern Oklahoma. During the many months of my seventy-mile-per-day bike treks, I could eat as much as I could hold and still lose weight and feel fantastic. This was a real bonus for a kid who had grown up quite overweight and with a very strong family history of diabetes. At that point in my life, my obesity and diabetes-prone genes were in complete harmony with my athletic lifestyle, and I looked and felt better than ever before, even though I probably packed away over 5,000 calories per day of wholesome food just to fuel my big commute. I still exercise most every day, but because I don't have the time or the inclination to ride a bike seventy miles per day, I have to watch my diet very closely or the "thrifty genes" take over and I gain weight readily.

A stark contrast to my lifestyle was seen in most of the patients who came to the hospital. It soon became clear to me that in whatever department I had to work, obesity and diabetes were the primary concern. Sedentary lifestyles and fast foods were a great curse to these people. In pediatrics, a substantial amount of time was spent counseling parents of overweight kids to keep their kids active and to get the junk food out of their diets. In obstetrics, gestational diabetes was almost the rule and seriously complicated pregnancies and deliveries were commonplace. In internal medicine, managing poorly controlled diabetes, premature heart disease, blindness, and end-stage kidney disease were routine. Sadly, in surgery, I became quite adept at performing amputations on so many diabetics who lost toes, feet, or legs to gangrene.

All in all, this was a moving experience in many ways and it motivated me to take lifestyle counseling, early diabetes detection, and aggressive diabetes management very seriously in all of my overweight patients. I am quite sure that I (now in my late forties would be a diabetic if I had let my "bad" genes dictate my fate, but I have avoided this by always paying close attention to my way of life and what goes in my mouth. Since my residency experiences were so vividly etched in my mind, I have been motivated to coach, exhort, counsel, and encourage hundreds of others to change the course of their lives and to spoil the dark plans that diabetes has for them. I now know with certainty that when it comes to diabetes, it is not just "all in the genes."

REDUCING THE EXPRESSION OF THE THRIFTY GENOTYPE

The key to both avoiding and reversing obesity is reducing the expression of the thrifty genotype. Can this actually be done? Definitely. That is what the Hunger Free Forever program is all about. Activation of the thrifty genotype is a lot like inviting a monster to come live inside your body. Once this monster is inside, it has a very powerful desire to take over—it wants to eat and it wants to grow. The monster that we are referring to is an accumulation of fat that resides in our abdominal cavity and surrounds our internal organs. This type of fat is also referred to as intra-abdominal fat and visceral adipose tissue.

The expression of the thrifty genotype and the hunger of the "monster" is largely the result of the impact of two opposing hormones secreted by fat cells in the abdomen: adiponectin, a compound that helps insulin work better, and resistin, a compound that blocks insulin's action. The levels of these fat-derived hormones go a long way in determining the body's sensitivity to the hormone insulin. Fortunately, our program reestablishes the proper ration of adiponectin to resistin and thus provides a key mechanism to improving the sensitivity to insulin, thereby reducing the expression of the thrifty genotype. And, as we will continually stress, improving the body's sensitivity to insulin is the key goal in breaking the weight-gain cycle, getting appetite under control, and allowing for maintenance of your ideal body weight.

CHAPTER SUMMARY

- Obesity can be calculated by determining your body mass index (BMI) or body fat percentage.
- Obesity is now the major cause of mortality in the United States.
- Obesity is emerging as a worldwide problem due to incorporation of the American diet and lifestyle.
- The increase in obesity rates in the United States parallels the rise in the intake of refined sugars like high fructose corn syrup (HFCS).
- Adopting a more Western diet is associated with an increased rate of obesity as well as virtually every other chronic disease.
- The presence of the "thrifty genotype" helps protect against starvation during famine, but increases the likelihood of developing obesity.
- The Hunger Free Forever program effectively prevents the expression of the thrifty genotype and allows you to achieve and maintain your ideal body weight.

2

THE SEVEN KEYS TO
HUNGER-FREE WEIGHT LOSS

Diets don't work. It is an undeniable fact. All of our weight-loss patients have tried various diets and have either failed to lose weight or have gained all the lost weight back and more. They are not alone. The statistics from the National Institutes of Health tell us that 98 percent of people who lose weight by dieting end up gaining it back within five years. And 90 percent of those people gain back more weight than they lost. Based upon these statistics, one could actually conclude that dieting is a significant contributor to obesity in the United States.

Diets fail because they result in an increased appetite drive as you lose weight, making it harder to resist temptation as time goes on. They also result in muscle loss, which lowers your metabolic rate, causing more of your extra calories to turn into fat. Most important, diets don't help you to make changes that you can live with for the rest of your life, so you tend to drift back gradually to your old habits.

The reason why people continue to go on diets even though the chances of success are so "slim" is simple: to do otherwise is contrary the conventional wisdom that an overweight person must lose weight by just eating less and exercising more. This "fact" is highlighted in every book about weight loss, but what the statistics on weight-loss success prove is that this notion of eating less and exercising more is far easier said than done. In fact, none of the diet programs from past and present have really done any good. We have more fat Americans than ever before.

While it is true that achieving weight loss is just about burning more calories than you consume, the reality is that it has been impossible for the dieter to achieve this goal—until now. The reason for failure prior to the Hunger Free Forever program comes down to a basic fact: Eating less and exercising more is impossible to accomplish in an overweight person when their appetite is out of control. With all of those powerful signals to eat, the dieter is virtually powerless to correct their bad habits and lose weight sensibly. However, by turning the hunger switch off, you are able to gain control of your appetite and actually achieve your weight-loss goals whether you follow our dietary plan or create your own.

WHY THE HUNGER FREE FOREVER PROGRAM IS DIFFERENT FROM GOING ON A DIET

Like a hungry bear before hibernation, it gets hungrier as it gets heavier, and as you gain weight, that weight gain actually promotes a magnification of your appetite, an increase in food cravings, and a reduced sense of satiety when you limit yourself to moderate-calorie food portions. It takes a lot to make the monster feel satisfied.

As discussed briefly in chapter 1, the principal source of this increase in appetite comes about from biochemical and hormonal changes that occur with an increase in internal belly fat (visceral adipose tissue) that occurs as you gain weight. As well, your eating habits, when unhealthy or based on poor food choices, become learned behaviors that form fixed patterns inside your brain, that will drive you to eat excessive amounts of the wrong kinds of foods, and can even evolve into obsessive or addictive behaviors that are very difficult to change.

So how can the Hunger Free Forever program help? First, we start by helping you achieve satiety and victory over your appetite. When our patients are able to get their appetite under control, it makes weight loss nearly effortless and allows them to adjust their eating habits so they can finally reach their weight-loss goals. Unlike popular diets that result in significant loss of lean body mass, the Hunger Free Forever program is most often accompanied by an increase in lean body mass and preservation of metabolic rate. The weight that does come off is fat, not muscle.

Second, we reestablish your body's sensitivity to insulin. When insulin sensitivity is restored, more nutrients enter muscle cells after each meal, making fewer calories available to fat cells and more calories available to give you energy and heat. Sensitivity to insulin is established by stabilizing blood sugar levels. After-meal blood sugar surges and hypoglycemic symptoms are eliminated within days of starting this program, resulting in a remarkable reduction in food cravings, and as a result, excess calories can be eliminated without discomfort.

Third, in addition to reducing appetite, eliminating food cravings, improving insulin sensitivity, and stabilizing blood sugar, we help people to identify the bad habits that are sabotaging their weight-loss efforts and then help them to understand how these behaviors can be painlessly modified and gradually replaced with habits that promote ideal weight. We also teach people how to accept these healthy lifestyle changes as a permanent way of life rather than just a temporary discipline while they are "on a diet." Even though many of these changes are based on common sense—like not skipping breakfast, eating more slowly, and avoiding sugary drinks—the only way to make healthy dietary changes a permanent way of life is to provide people with a long-term solution that will reduce their appetite and eliminate unhealthy food cravings so that they are not driven back to their old behaviors. When addictive and excessive food cravings are gone, good sense can rule and a person can follow the healthy changes we recommend with little sacrifice and no discomfort. Then, we focus on the importance of learning to set positive goal statements and visualizing success to realize your long-term weight-loss goals.

We have labeled the key features of our program the Seven Keys to Hunger-Free Weight Loss. While each of these keys is critical to long-term success, the most important by far is achieving high satiety and controlling the appetite. Each of these keys will be discussed fully in subsequent chapters where you will gain an in-depth appreciation of just how interconnected they are in controlling the appetite and taming the monster within.

The Seven Keys to Hunger-Free Weight Loss

1. Restore Blood Sugar Stability
2. Develop Eating Strategies for High Satiety
3. Transform Your Habits, Transform Your Life
4. Reduce the Effects of Stress and Cortisol
5. Tone Your Muscles, Train Your Heart
6. Rev Up Your Metabolism
7. Program Yourself for Success

Understanding Appetite

Oxygen, food, and water are the three principal things that we need to remain alive. We don't think much about oxygen until we hold our breath and experience an overwhelming desire to breathe again. Likewise, if we are deprived of food, the body has powerful mechanisms to keep us interested in and seeking after nourishment. Throughout history, reproduction and survival have often favored those humans who had a very strong desire to eat. As we have learned about the "thrifty genotype," those of us who have had to struggle with our weight can probably thank our ancestors for giving us such a remarkable ability to gain it.

Even though some people possess the thrifty genotype (see chapter 1) or seem to be endowed with a much heartier appetite than others, all of us eat when we sense an inner need for food. We tend to eat until we sense a feeling of fullness or satiety that tells us that we have had enough. The ultimate success of any weight-loss strategy comes down to helping people learn how to achieve a sense of satiety with fewer calories than their body desires or needs.

Is Your Appetite in Overdrive?

People without weight problems benefit from a complex and properly working system of appetite control composed of compounds that circulate in the blood such as various hormones, peptides, neurotransmitters, and glucose, all of which are sensed and acted upon by the brain. People of normal weight don't tend to experience frequent and unhealthy food cravings, and they usually feel hungry at appropriate times. They are also inclined to feel satisfied when they have eaten modest-sized food portions that don't promote weight gain.

Unfortunately, in overweight and obese individuals, this complex system of appetite control becomes altered. As a result, they possess an increased appetite drive along with frequent and excessive food cravings. They become more sensitive to both internal and external signals to eat, and they are less able to experience a strong sense of satiety when they have eaten adequate amounts of food.

Resetting Appetite Control

As we discussed in chapter 1, in more primitive times the tendency to pack on the weight when food was overly abundant would have had survival benefits when famine was around the corner. Today, with a plentiful and abundant food supply, we never experience the famine and as a result our physiology is stuck in the fat-storing mode with an overactive appetite. If you want to get your weight under control and remain at an ideal weight for life, you must get this unhealthy appetite control system restored to a healthy state where you are free from excessive food cravings and an appetite in overdrive. That is exactly what the Hunger Free Forever program has been shown to do.

In hundreds of cases, we have witnessed how this program has helped people who struggled with their weight for years and failed at diets over and over again. The big difference with the Hunger Free Forever program is that people find themselves finally liberated from excessive hunger pangs and are then able to adjust their eating behaviors and reduce their portion sizes without any discomfort.

CHAPTER SUMMARY

- Statistics tell us that 98 percent of people who lose weight by dieting end up gaining it back within five years. And 90 percent of those people gain back more weight than they lost.
- Eating less and exercising more is impossible to accomplish for an overweight person when their appetite is out of control.
- Weight gain promotes magnification of appetite, increase in food cravings, and reduced sense of satiety.

- The fundamental difference with our program is that we start by helping people to achieve satiety and victory over their appetite.
- The center of the goal of improving satiety is rapidly restoring the body's sensitivity to the hormone insulin and the ability to regulate blood sugar.
- The only way to make healthy dietary changes a permanent way of life is to provide people with a long-term solution that will reduce their appetite and eliminate unhealthy food cravings.

3

RESTORE BLOOD
SUGAR STABILITY

Using breakthrough technology, we have discovered that one of the absolute keys to achieving effective weight loss and long-term weight control is to maintain glucose or blood sugar levels within a very narrow range. The notion that optimal blood sugar control plays an important role in the regulation of appetite is not new. What is new is that we were the first to conduct landmark research demonstrating that frequent and rapid swings in blood sugar underly the magnified appetite and frequent food cravings so typical of individuals who are struggling with their weight. We refer to this unstable state of blood sugar control as "increased glycemic (blood sugar) volatility."

We have seen clearly that increased glycemic volatility is an abnormality that can be demonstrated in almost every person with a weight problem. It is highly correlated to their inability to lose weight and keep it off. In contrast, our program utilizes a combination of therapeutic products and dietary changes that brings about a rapid reduction in glycemic volatility and a marked stabilization in blood sugar. Reducing blood sugar volatility and improving the action of insulin is one of the key reasons our program is so successful in achieving effective and permanent weight loss. When blood sugar is highly stable around the clock, appetite is reduced and undesirable food cravings are remarkably diminished, making weight loss and long-term weight maintenance well within the reach of most people.

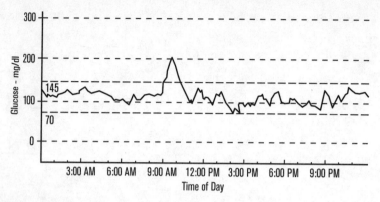

Figure 3.1. Overweight Adult Before Weight Loss Demonstrating Elevated Blood Sugar (Glycemic) Volatility.

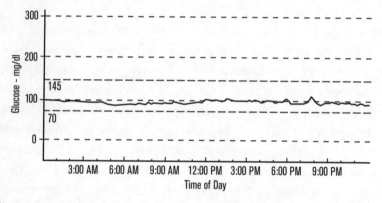

Figure 3.2. Healthy (Nonvolatile) 24-hour Continuous Blood Sugar in an Overweight Adult Six Weeks into the Hunger Free Forever Program.

A GLUCOSE PRIMER

While fat is the preferred energy source in most tissues, the brain is critically dependent upon glucose as its energy source. If blood glucose levels were to drop below a certain minimum value, death would occur in a few seconds. Therefore, there are a lot of very sophisticated feedback and control mechanisms that ensure the brain has a constant, steady supply of glucose to prevent you from simply running out and falling over dead.

The majority of glucose in the body is derived from dietary carbohydrates. There are two groups of carbohydrates, simple and complex. Simple carbohydrates, or sugars, are naturally found in fruits and vegetables, but most of the simple sugars consumed in developed countries are in the form of refined sugar like sucrose (white sugar). Complex carbohydrates include starch and other, larger carbohydrate molecules.

When high sugar, or low fiber, starchy foods are eaten in excess, blood sugar levels rise quickly, producing a strain on blood sugar control. The body responds to the rise in blood glucose levels after meals by secreting insulin, a hormone produced by the beta cells of the pancreas (a small gland that resides at the base of the stomach). Insulin lowers blood glucose by increasing the rate that glucose is taken up by cells throughout the body. Declines in blood glucose, as occur during fasting or exercise, cause the release of glucagon, another hormone produced by the pancreas. Glucagon stimulates the release of glucose stored in the muscles and liver as glycogen. If blood sugar levels fall sharply or if a person is angry or frightened, it may result in the release of epinephrine (Adrenalin) and corticosteroids (cortisol) by the adrenal glands. These hormones provide quicker breakdown of stored glucose for extra energy during a crisis or increased need.

Ideally, these mechanisms are effective in keeping blood sugar levels within a very narrow range. Unfortunately, a great deal of Americans stress these control mechanisms through diet and lifestyle. As a result, obesity, diabetes, and other disorders of blood sugar regulation are among the most common diseases of modern society.

THE IMPORTANCE OF CARBOHYDRATES IN WEIGHT MANAGEMENT

Low-carb and no-carb diets have enjoyed tremendous popularity as a weight-loss strategy. Often they can produce quick and dramatic results, but those short-term benefits are outweighed by rebound weight gain. When the body is starved for carbohydrates, it will initially derive glucose by breaking down the storage form of glucose (glycogen) stored in the muscles and liver and releasing it into the

(continued on next page)

bloodstream as glucose. If you were completely without food, there is enough glycogen stored in your muscles and liver to supply your bloodstream with glucose for about two days (much less if you are exercising during starvation). If starvation continues after this stored glycogen is gone, the body will sacrifice tissues and organs containing protein, and that protein is broken down into glucose by the liver so that blood glucose never goes below the level required to sustain life. In addition, the brain switches gears a bit and is able to burn not only glucose for energy, but also compounds known as ketones. This energy source is produced in the liver from fatty acids. Ketones have a strong characteristic odor and are the reason many people following a low-carb diet experience bad breath similar to the breath of alcohol intoxication.

Is ketosis necessary for weight loss? Absolutely not, and while ketosis is usually not dangerous (though it can be life-threatening if severe, especially in a diabetic), it is certainly not a particularly healthful state. In addition, one of the major problems with a low-carb diet or even a very low–calorie diet is that they inevitably produce a loss of significant amounts of muscle mass. The muscle is sacrificed in order to provide the dieter with a constant supply of blood sugar. In fact, if you lose weight through fasting or other forms of severe dieting, a significant proportion of the weight loss will be in the form of water (each molecule of glycogen binds six water molecules) and muscle mass. This sort of weight loss will significantly lower your metabolic rate and reduce the primary fat-burning furnace in the body, lean muscle mass, thereby setting you up for serious weight gain later on.

Insulin and Blood Sugar Control

Proper blood sugar control is dependent upon the action of insulin. You can think of insulin as a key that opens the door of the cell, letting in glucose to feed it. Around the clock, the pancreas secretes a small amount of insulin that allows necessary amounts of glucose to enter into cells to keep them alive and energized. After a meal, as the bloodstream becomes flooded with glucose, a large pulse of insulin is released from the pancreas, resulting in a significant increase in the uptake of glucose into muscles and other organs. In this way, the sugar in the blood is quickly transferred to organs, energizing them and keeping blood sugar from rising too high.

Unfortunately, when you start gaining weight, particularly when you gain internal belly fat (visceral adipose tissue), substances are secreted from the visceral adipose tissue that promote insulin resistance, a condition in which insulin is released but no longer works as effectively as it should. Insulin, as a molecule, is still the same, but the cells throughout the body lose some of their ability to sense and respond properly to it.

Because elevated blood sugar is so harmful, the body works hard to keep blood sugar normal as insulin resistance develops. It does this by releasing higher than normal amounts of insulin around the clock and particularly after meals. In fact, if insulin levels did not rise substantially as insulin resistance developed, diabetes would inevitably occur in the early stages of insulin resistance. In most cases, these high levels of insulin fend off diabetes for some time, but have several implications for those who are now living with a weight problem.

Glucose: A Double-Edged Sword

We have stressed the importance of glucose in supplying energy to the brain, and the fact that if blood sugar levels drop too low, you die. The same is true if blood sugar levels go too high, though it is a longer, more insidious death. Because glucose is fuel for your body, in many ways it is like gasoline for your car. If you run out of glucose, your body will "quit" just like when your car runs out of gas. Likewise, whenever your blood glucose levels are elevated, it creates a toxic mess just as it would if you spilled gasoline when you were filling your car. In optimal health, the body maintains very tight control over blood glucose levels and it works very hard to keep those levels within a narrow range.

When blood glucose levels surge too high, excessive glucose cannot be readily taken up by cells. It begins to bind to various body proteins and other molecules, changing their structure and creating physiological chaos. These "sugar-coated molecules" are called "advanced glycosylated end products" and their accumulation is considered to be one of the principal factors that lead to accelerated aging and, eventually, death. Excessive glycosylation has many adverse effects: inactivation of enzymes, inhibition of regulatory molecule binding, and the formation of abnormal protein structures, to name a few. Of course, diabetes is characterized by persistent and repeated elevations in blood glucose and glycosylated proteins. As a result, it provides the grave example of the damage that can be produced when blood sugar levels get too high and there is excessive glycosylation.

Major Complications of Diabetes

- Heart disease and stroke: Adults with diabetes have death rates from cardiovascular disease about two to four times higher than adults without diabetes.
- High blood pressure: About 75 percent of adults with diabetes have high blood pressure.
- Blindness: Diabetes is the leading cause of blindness among adults.
- Kidney disease: Diabetes is the leading reason why people need to go on dialysis, accounting for 43 percent of new cases.
- Nervous system disease: About 60 to 70 percent of people with diabetes have mild to severe forms of nervous system damage. Severe forms of diabetic nerve disease are a major contributing cause of lower-extremity amputations.
- Amputations: More than 60 percent of lower-limb amputations in the United States occur among people with diabetes.
- Periodontal disease: Almost one third of people with diabetes have severe periodontal (gum) disease.
- Pain: Many diabetics fall victim to chronic pain due to conditions such as arthritis, neuropathy, circulatory insufficiency, or fibromyalgia.
- Depression is a common accompaniment of diabetes. Clinical depression can often begin to occur even years before diabetes is fully evident. As well, depression is difficult to treat in poorly controlled diabetics.
- Autoimmune disorders: Thyroid disease, inflammatory arthritis, and other diseases of the immune system commonly add to the suffering of diabetes.

THE PROBLEM IS NOT A LACK OF INSULIN

At our clinic, we measure insulin levels in most of our weight-loss patients. We commonly discover their fasting insulin levels to be two to three times the normal value, even in many who are only modestly overweight. Even though fasting blood sugar levels or glucose tolerance tests are "normal" in many of these people, we consider those with evidence of insulin resistance to be "diabetics in training." Research suggests that many of these individuals will eventually become diabetics when their pancreas finally tires and is unable to produce the massive amount of insulin required to keep their blood sugar out of the diabetic range. Moreover, we now realize that insulin resistance—even if diabetes never develops—brings with it a whole host of serious health problems. Restoring insulin sensitivity is the only real answer to this dilemma and one of the principal goals of the Hunger Free Forever program.

Our program is especially beneficial if you have type 2 diabetes. Roughly 90 percent of the 18 million American with diabetes have type 2 diabetes. Type 2 diabetes is intricately linked to obesity, in particular to increased visceral adipose tissue (belly fat). While in type 1 diabetes there is insufficient insulin production, requiring daily insulin therapy, in type 2 diabetes insulin levels are typically initially elevated, indicating a loss of sensitivity to insulin by the cells of the body. With the Hunger Free Forever program we help to restore insulin sensitivity, thereby potentially reversing the signs and symptoms of type 2 diabetes.

ARE YOU A DIABETIC IN TRAINING?

Pre-diabetes, also called "impaired glucose tolerance," is a condition that occurs when a person's blood glucose levels are higher than normal but not high enough for a diagnosis of type 2 diabetes. There are almost as many people in the United States with pre-diabetes (about 16 million) as there are diabetics. Although many of these people are reassured by their doctors or told that they just have "a touch of dia-

(continued on next page)

betes," research increasingly indicates that impaired glucose tolerance, even if diabetes never fully manifests, is accompanied by
serious health risks and it should be treated carefully.

Many people with impaired glucose tolerance fulfill other criteria of what is known as the metabolic syndrome. This condition,
originally referred to as "syndrome X" by Stanford University endo-
crinologist Gerald Reaven, M.D., refers to a cluster of metabolic risk
factors that includes:

- Central obesity (excessive fat tissue in and around the abdomen)
  as demonstrated by a greater waist-to-hip ratio
- Low levels of HDL cholesterol:
  - Men: Less than 40 mg/dl
  - Women: Less than 50 mg/dl
- Fasting blood triglycerides greater than or equal to 150mg/dl
- Elevated blood pressure (130/85mmHg or higher)
- Insulin resistance (the body can't properly use insulin or blood
  glucose), as demonstrated by the presence of pre-diabetes (glucose
  levels between 101 and 125mg/dl)

The metabolic syndrome is a serious health issue, because people who
have it are at increased risk for coronary artery disease, other diseases
related to plaque buildup in artery walls (e.g., stroke and peripheral
vascular disease), and type 2 diabetes. The presence of four or more of
the above criteria is associated with a two and a half times greater risk
of having a heart attack or stroke and a nearly twenty-five times greater
risk of developing diabetes.

It is estimated that about 60 million adults in the United States
meet the criteria for the metabolic syndrome. The metabolic syndrome—as well as type 2 diabetes, pre-diabetes, and obesity—can be
viewed as different facets of the same disease, having the same underlying dietary, lifestyle, and genetic causes. The bottom line is that the
human body was simply not designed to handle the amount of refined
sugar, white flour, salt, saturated fat, and other harmful food components that many people in the United States and other Western coun-

tries—especially those who live a sedentary lifestyle—consume. The result is the emergence of metabolic syndrome and type 2 diabetes with all of their accompanying health risks.

RECOMMENDATIONS FOR THE EARLY DETECTION OF DIABETES AND OTHER DISEASES

Item	Recommendation
Wellness checkup	A wellness checkup is recommended every year for children up to 18 years of age; every three years for people age 19–40, and every year for people age 40 or older. This exam should include health counseling and, depending on a person's age and sex, a complete physical exam and screening for diabetes, cancer, and heart disease. Laboratory assessment should include at the bare minimum a complete blood count (CBC); fasting blood glucose; and cholesterol levels (including LDL and HDL determination). We also recommend determining C-reactive protein (CRP) levels. The goal is keeping your CRP level below 1.0mg/L. (See chapter 7 for more information about C-reactive protein.)

Beginning at age 50, men and women should follow one of the examination schedules below:

- A fecal occult blood test every year and a flexible sigmoidoscopy every five years.
- A colonoscopy every ten years.
- A double-contrast barium enema every five to ten years.

A digital rectal exam (including prostate exam in men) should be done at the same time as sigmoidoscopy, colonoscopy, or double-contrast barium enema.

People who have a family history of colon cancer should talk with a doctor about a different testing schedule.

(continued on next page)

RECOMMENDATIONS FOR THE EARLY DETECTION OF DIABETES AND OTHER DISEASES *(continued)*

Item	Recommendation
Special exams for women	All women 18 and older should have an annual Pap test and pelvic examination. They should also have an annual clinical breast examination by a health care professional and should perform monthly breast self-examinations. Women with a family history of cancer of the uterus should have a sample of endometrial tissue examined when menopause begins. Women 40 and older should also have an annual mammogram.
Special exams for men	To screen for prostate cancer, we recommend getting both the prostate-specific antigen (PSA) blood test and the digital rectal examination annually beginning at age 40, especially for men in high-risk groups, such as those with a strong familial predisposition, and African Americans.

Insulin Resistance, Weight Gain, and Appetite

Insulin itself is classified as an anabolic hormone. That means that it promotes growth of both muscle and fat in those who are insulin sensitive. Unfortunately, when insulin resistance develops, insulin continues to stimulate the growth of fat, but has little effect on muscle. Those who develop insulin resistance and its accompanying elevated insulin levels (hyperinsulinemia) have a hormonal tendency to deposit fat and lose muscle mass. In essence, when you are insulin resistant, your muscles are starved and your fat cells are overfed. Because of this, it is very difficult for fat to be burned efficiently when you are in an insulin-resistant state. Unless insulin sensitivity is restored, weight loss through dieting is an uphill battle at best and is impossible for most people.

It used to be thought that the brain was not affected by insulin. This belief was based upon a false assumption that there were no insulin receptors in the brain. However, insulin receptors have now been discovered in nearly every region of the brain, especially those regions in charge of controlling appetite. In insulin-sensitive people, a rise of insulin after meals results in a promotion of satiety through its action in the brain. However, in those with insulin resistance, even the excessive insulin levels experienced after meals no longer result in a significant sense of satiety.

In normal individuals, it has been shown that regions of the brain responsible for appetite regulation respond to after-meal elevations in insulin by significantly increasing their intake of glucose and, subsequently, increasing the metabolic activity in these regions. In particular, the brain regions most responsible for appetite, such as the hypothalamus, readily respond to insulin. This reaction to insulin results in a decrease in appetite and a sense of satiety. In contrast, those with insulin resistance have been shown to lack this increase in metabolic activity in these important brain regions following a significant rise in insulin levels. We now know that the brain becomes insulin resistant along with the rest of the body, and that this insulin resistance plays an important role in the loss of after-meal satiety that accompanies weight gain. Think of the appetite control center having an "off" button for appetite that will only respond to insulin. With insulin resistance, the appetite never really gets shut down.

Insulin Resistance and Blood Sugar Control

Obviously, one of the key abnormalities in insulin-resistant individuals is their loss of precise control over blood sugar. To a large extent because of their frequently increased blood sugar levels, these "diabetics in training" experience the same kinds of accelerated aging and tissue damage that occurs in diabetics, but at a slower pace. Cardiovascular disease, high blood pressure, liver disease, and kidney damage are just a few of the many complications that can arise from pre-diabetes. Importantly, for those who want to lose weight, this loss of precision control over blood sugar results in a significant increase in appetite.

When blood sugar surges after a meal in those with insulin resistance, it is accompanied by a massive release of insulin. This insulin does eventually activate insulin receptors to open up cells to glucose, and this glucose surge is usually followed by a rapid drop in blood sugar. As blood sugar plummets, the brain, pancreas, and liver sense this rapid drop and an emergency is declared, since extremely low blood sugar is potentially deadly. To prevent severe low blood sugar (hypoglycemia), hormones such as glucagon, epinephrine (Adrenalin), and cortisol are released, all of which promote the release of stored glycogen from the liver and muscles, and result in the synthesis of glucose from dietary or body protein. As a result, those with insulin resistance will experience food cravings as their blood sugar begins to drop. In essence, the brain is alarmed by any rapid drop in blood sugar, so it does everything it can to get you to reach for a quick sugar fix.

It has been known since the 1950s that a sudden decrease in blood sugar over a short period of time is a primary trigger for food cravings and eating, if food is readily available. Several experiments on both animals and humans support this so called "glucostatic theory" of appetite control. Although we know that the control of appetite is influenced by a whole orchestra of hormones, peptides, and neurotransmitters, glucose can still be considered a lead player and perhaps the conductor of this orchestra. Currently, we know that rapid and deep drops in blood sugar are particularly associated with very strong, and in some cases irresistible, urges to eat.

Do You Experience Symptoms of Hypoglycemia?

Sweating, weakness, dizziness, shakiness, and rapid heart rate are examples of symptoms of hypoglycemia (hypo = low; glycemia = blood sugar). Since the brain is critically dependent upon blood sugar as its primary fuel, when hypoglycemia becomes more severe, the brain is seriously affected. In such cases, symptoms of hypoglycemia can range from mild to severe and include such things as: headache, depression, anxiety, irritability, blurred vision, excessive sweating, mental confusion, incoherent speech, bizarre behavior, lack of coordination, and later, if blood sugar goes below critical levels, convulsions, coma, and even death. Insulin- or medication-treated diabetics need to develop a keen awareness of hypoglycemia because serious hypoglycemia episodes can be dangerous. Unfortunately, the bodies of many diabetics become less sensitive to the initial adrenaline-related signs of impending hypoglycemia over time (sweating, weakness, rapid heart rate, etc.). These individuals must develop an ability to monitor subtleties of their brain function instead in an effort to achieve good blood sugar control and avoid catastrophic hypoglycemic episodes.

What about less severe symptoms of hypoglycemia? Great controversy has arisen over this concept. The medical profession has resisted the notion that people without diabetes can experience significant hypoglycemia except in rare cases of insulin-producing tumors of the pancreas or medical conditions such as alcoholism. Many nondiabetics indeed experience symptoms suggestive of hypoglycemia. One to three hours after meals, they begin to feel weak, shaky, and dizzy, and experience strong food cravings, especially for sweets. Many of the same people know that if they eat something—particularly high carbohydrate foods—when they experience these symptoms that the symptoms usually improve or resolve within a few minutes. Many have also learned that if they avoid sugary or starchy foods and eat meals high in protein along with frequent high-protein snacks, they can reduce or avoid these symptoms significantly. All of this does indeed sound like hypoglycemia; however, when their blood sugar is checked during these episodes, it is *uncommon* for it to be in the significantly or dangerously hypoglycemic range. Although many of these people have accepted the concept that they suffer from hypoglycemia and may even refer to themselves as "hypoglycemics," they seldom find a medical doctor who will support this diagnosis.

From our research using continuous blood glucose monitors with our patients, we believe that most of these individuals actually experience rapidly dropping blood sugar with or without mild to moderate hypoglycemia. This is a direct result of insulin resistance and a loss of precise control over blood sugar. In people who are prone to such symptoms, these uncomfortable experiences occur more frequently and with greater magnitude when they eat foods that have a high glycemic impact.

Elevated Glycemic Volatility

We have found that even if their blood sugar never drops below normal, many individuals experience blood sugar surges after meals followed by rapidly dropping blood sugar. It is during the time that the

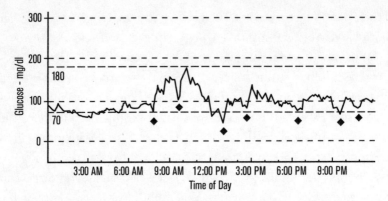

Figure 3.3. In this case, black diamonds represent times when the patient feels "hypoglycemic" and then responds by eating. Each time represents an episode of rapidly dropping blood sugar, but only two occasions (while awake) are actual hypoglycemic episodes (below 70mg/dl). Elevated glycemic volatility with rapid drops in blood sugar explains most "hypoglycemic" symptoms in nondiabetics and it is even more commonly associated with food cravings or "hunger pangs."

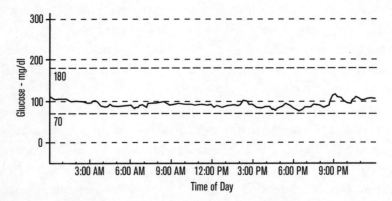

Figure 3.4. Same patient four weeks into the Hunger Free Forever program. Hypoglycemic symptoms and excessive food cravings are now resolved.

blood sugar is dropping rapidly that hormones like adrenaline and cortisol are released, creating weakness, agitation, and shakiness. The hunger pangs and brain fog that accompany a drop in blood sugar probably result from decreased brain metabolism as well as glucosensory brain receptors detecting this rapidly dropping glucose and then responding by sending out strong signals that it is time to eat. Hypo-glycemia is not the best term to describe this condition, since most often blood sugar levels do not go below normal values. Instead, we call this condition of rapidly fluctuating blood sugar "elevated glyce-mic volatility" and we have good reason to believe that elevated glyce-mic volatility is at the heart of most weight problems. What we have discovered is that rapidly fluctuating blood sugar levels are generally related to some degree of insulin resistance and made worse by wrong food choices (more than a moderate amount of high glycemic impact foods).

ARE YOU RIDING THE BLOOD SUGAR ROLLER COASTER?

Do any of the following apply to you?

- My waist circumference is larger than my hips.
- It is difficult for me to lose weight.
- I crave sweets.
- I feel much better after I eat.
- I am very irritable if I miss a meal.
- Sometimes I feel a bit spacey and disconnected.
- I have elevated blood sugar or triglyceride levels.
- I get anxious for no apparent reason.
- I wake up often during the night.
- I feel hungry all of the time.
- I often get very sleepy in the afternoon.

We have found that these symptoms and signs are very common in our patients with blood sugar volatility. How do we know they really have blood sugar volatility? Our research center was the first in the world to utilize a remarkable new technology as a tool for understanding the increased appetite and frequent food cravings so typical of individuals who are struggling with their weight, and to then use this technology in helping overweight and obese people succeed in their weight-loss efforts. The technology, known as the continuous glucose monitoring system (CGMS) from Medtronic MiniMed, has provided an amazing window through which we can view an overweight person's blood sugar on a continuous basis.

The CGMS is an electronic diagnostic system that requires the insertion of a sensing catheter under the skin of the abdomen. The sensing catheter contains a miniaturized electronic device that measures blood sugar and then sends this information every few seconds to a pager-sized computer module worn on the patient's belt for up to one week. The portable computer module translates and records blood sugar data, which can then be downloaded to the doctor's computer. A graph showing the average blood sugar reading every five minutes (288 blood sugar readings per day) can then be generated and studied in relationship to food intake, appetite, food cravings, hypoglycemic symptoms, medication, and exercise.

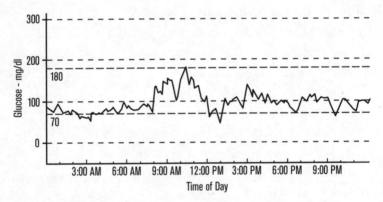

Figure 3.5. Continuous glucose graph over 24 hours in typical overweight, nondiabetic patient before the Hunger Free Forever program. Patient has elevated glycemic volatility (she is on the blood sugar roller coaster). Monitoring for several days showed that this was her consistent pattern even when she ate healthy food. Frequent food cravings were reported to occur at times when blood sugar rapidly dropped over short periods of time. This amounted to several significant food cravings per day. Feelings of hypoglycemia also occurred when blood sugar dropped rapidly, even when blood sugar was in the normal range. (Note: normal blood sugar is between 70 and 100 mg/dl. This patient was spending most of the day outside this ideal range.)

Using the CGMS, we have discovered that most people with weight problems go through their days with remarkably fluctuating blood sugar or increased glycemic volatility. We now believe that getting people off the blood sugar roller coaster is essential to helping them successfully lose weight and keep it off. We have seen how this glycemic volatility is worsened with higher glycemic impact foods, but it is first fundamentally related to insulin resistance and a loss of precise control over blood sugar. Figure 3.5 and Figure 3.6 show what this data looks like before and after our program, respectively.

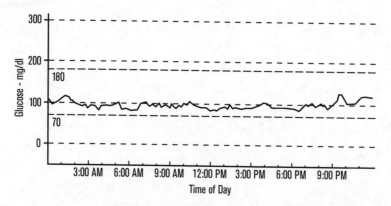

Figure 3.6. Continuous glucose graph over 24 hours in same patient four weeks into Hunger Free Forever program. Patient now has nearly normalized glycemic volatility. Appetite and food cravings have dramatically diminished. Hypoglycemic symptoms no longer occur at all. As well, patient has more energy and mental clarity. Weight loss is progressing on target and with no discomfort. This type of change is very typical with the Hunger Free Forever program and it dramatically illustrates the remarkable changes that occur with this program.

With the CGMS, we have also diagnosed many people with diabetes who failed to demonstrate diabetes with the typical diagnostic tests. Since early recognition and treatment are of critical importance in the outcome of diabetes, we believe the CGMS could play a vital role in the prevention and early detection of diabetes.

HYPOGLYCEMIA: A HISTORICAL AND MODERN PERSPECTIVE

Both of us became interested in nutrition in the 1970s. At that time, hypoglycemia was a popular self-diagnosis. There were a number of popular books, such as *Sugar Blues* by William Duffy, *Hope for Hypoglycemia* by Broda Barnes, and *Sweet and Dangerous* by John Yudkin, which fueled this public interest. In these books, the dangers of too much sugar in the diet were clearly spelled out. Yet since those books were published, the per capita of sugar consumption has risen dramatically. The average American now consumes over 100 pounds of sucrose and 40 pounds of corn syrup each year. This sugar addiction probably plays a major role in the high prevalence of poor health and chronic disease in the United States.

Research in the past three decades has provided an ever-increasing amount of new information on the role that both refined carbohydrates (sugar, high fructose corn syrup, and low-fiber starchy foods) and faulty blood sugar control play in many disease processes. New terminology and descriptions, such as the metabolic syndrome and impaired glucose tolerance, are now used to describe the complex hormonal fluxes that are largely a result of the ingestion of too many refined carbohydrates. However, what research has failed to demonstrate consistently is that the symptoms of hypoglycemia actually correlate to low blood sugar levels. What our research with the CGMS has shown is that the symptoms of hypoglycemia can occur simply as a result of rapidly falling blood sugar levels, and not solely as a result of the blood sugar level ever dropping below normal. This finding helps explain why symptoms of hypoglycemia in the past correlated so poorly with actual blood sugar levels. It is not the level, but rather *how fast the drop* that is important.

GETTING OFF THE BLOOD SUGAR ROLLER COASTER

If you are riding the blood sugar roller coaster, it will be nearly impossible to lose weight. Frequent fluctuations in blood sugar, particularly when blood sugar rapidly drops in a short period of time, can result in serious food cravings even when your body has no real need for additional calories. If these events occur dozens of times per day, you are likely to give in and snack or drink sugary drinks, and those snacks and beverages will likely be loaded with calories. In the face of these food cravings, if you use sheer willpower and hold off until your next meal, your appetite will be in overdrive and it is likely that you will eat too much of the wrong thing. Eating when your brain is sending out powerful signals to eat is not a good way to control your food choices, portion sizes, or speed of eating.

We have seen over and over again that reducing glycemic volatility is the single most important change that will make weight-loss efforts pleasant, comfortable, and effective. We have worked with hundreds of people who have tried and failed to lose weight through dieting. We have seen the remarkable transformation that occurs in these people when their blood sugar becomes stabilized and they no longer have to struggle with frequent food cravings and an appetite in overdrive. If you want to lose weight and keep it off for life, take the following steps to get off the blood sugar roller coaster and onto the blood sugar superhighway instead. The five key steps to reduce blood sugar volatility include:

1. Following a low glycemic load diet.
2. Increasing your intake of dietary fiber and eating adequate protein throughout the day.
3. Taking PGX with every meal.
4. Engaging in a regular exercise program.
5. Taking a high potency multiple vitamin with chromium.

Following a Low-Glycemic Load Diet: The Glycemic Index and Glycemic Load

Every food affects blood sugar differently. You must become familiar with how foods affect your blood sugar and begin to make sensible food choices, preferring foods that have a lower impact on blood sugar. This does not mean that you should avoid carbohydrates (as the Atkins Diet or the South Beach Diet prescribes) or that you need some special ratio of carbohydrates to protein and fat (as the Zone Diet prescribes). We have found that blood sugar can be completely stabilized in nondiabetics and improved dramatically in diabetics when significant amounts of healthy carbohydrates are included in the diet. The key is to choose carbohydrates wisely and to consume modest portion sizes. Two tools to help you in this goal are the glycemic index and glycemic load.

The glycemic index (GI) is a numerical scale used to indicate how fast and how high a particular food raises blood glucose (blood sugar) levels. There are two versions of the GI, one based on a standard of comparison that uses glucose scored as 100; the other is based on white bread. Foods are tested against the results of the selected standard. Refined sugars, white flour products, and other sources of simple sugars are quickly absorbed into the bloodstream, causing a rapid rise in blood sugar. In response, the body boosts secretion of insulin by the pancreas. High-sugar junk food diets definitely lead to poor blood sugar regulation, obesity, and ultimately type 2 diabetes. And, because of the stress on the body that they cause, including secreting too much insulin, they can also promote the growth of cancer and increase the risk of heart disease. Our simple recommendation? Don't eat "junk foods," and pay attention to the glycemic index of food that you eat.

The GI in quite useful, but since it doesn't tell how much carbohydrates is in a typical serving of a particular food, another tool is needed. That is where glycemic load comes in. The glycemic load (GL) is a relatively new way to assess the impact of carbohydrate consumption. It takes the glycemic index into account, but gives a more complete picture of the effect that a particular food has on blood sugar levels based on how much carbohydrate you actually eat in serving. A GL of 20 or more is high, a GL of 11 to 19 inclusive is medium, and a GL of 10 or less is low. For example, let's take a look at beets, a food with a high GI but low GL. Although the carbohydrate in beets has a high GI, there isn't a lot of it, so a typical serving of cook beets has a glycemic load that is very low, about 5. Thus, as long as you eat a reasonable portion of a low–glycemic load food, the impact on blood sugar is acceptable, even if the food is high in its GI.

To help you design your diet, we have provided a list of the glycemic index, fiber content, and glycemic load of common foods in appendix B. In essence, foods that are mostly water (e.g., apple or

CLASSIFICATION OF FOODS BY GLYCEMIC INDEX SCORES

Fruits and Vegetables		Grains, nuts, legumes	
Very High	Medium	Very High	Medium
None	Cantaloupe	Refined sugar	Brown rice
	Grapes	Most cold cereals	Oatmeal
	Orange	(e.g., Grape Nuts,	Pasta
	Orange juice	corn flakes, Raisin	Peas
	Peach	Bran, etc.)	Pita bread
	Pineapple	Rice Cakes	Pinto beans
	Watermelon	Granola	Rye bread
			Whole-grain breads
			Yams
High	**Low**	**High**	**Low**
Banana	Green beans	Bagel	Lentils
Raisins	Green pepper	Bread (white flour)	Nuts
Beets	Lettuce	Carrots	Seeds
Apple	Mushrooms	Corn	
Apricot	Onions	Granola Bar	
Asparagus	Plums	Kidney beans	
Broccoli	Spinach	Muffin (bran)	
Brussels sprouts	Strawberries	Potato	
Cauliflower	Tomato	Pretzel	
Celery	Zucchini	White rice	
Cherries		Tortilla	
Cucumber			
Grapefruit			

watermelon), fiber (e.g., beet or carrot), or air (e.g., popcorn) will not cause a steep rise in your blood sugar even if their glycemic index is high, as long as you exercise moderation in portion sizes. We recommend keeping the glycemic load for any three-hour period less than 20. For more information on planning a low-glycemic load diet, see chapter 10.

EXAMPLES OF GI, GL, AND INSULIN STRESS SCORE OF SELECTED FOODS

Food	GI	GL	Insulin stress (or glycemic impact)
Carrots, cooked, ½ cup	49	1.5	low
Peach, fresh, 1 large	42	3	low
Beets, cooked, ½ cup	64	3	low
Watermelon, ½ cup	72	4	low
Whole-wheat bread, 1 slice	69	9.6	low
Baked potato, medium	93	14	medium
Brown rice, cooked, 1 cup	50	16	medium
Banana, raw, 1 medium	55	17.6	medium
Spaghetti, white, cooked, 1 cup	41	23	high
White rice, cooked, 1 cup	72	26	high
Grape Nuts, ½ cup	71	33	very high
Soft drinks, 375 ml	68	34.7	very high

Avoid junk food and hidden sources of empty calories

According to the third National Health and Nutrition Examination Survey, which studied eating habits among 15,000 American adults, one third of the average diet in this country is made up of unhealthy foods, including potato chips, crackers, salted snack foods, candy, gum, fried fast food, and soft drinks. These items offer little in terms of protein, fiber, vitamins, or minerals. What they do offer is lots of "empty calories" in the form of sugar, white flour, and fat. They fill you up with extra calories and leave you with little interest in the foods that give your body a fighting chance to prevent heart disease, cancer, and other diseases.

How can you make healthier food choices and avoid the pitfalls of junk food? Here are a few guidelines:

- Read labels carefully. If sugar, flour (other than whole-grain flour), fat, or salt are among the first three ingredients listed, it is probably not a good option.

- Be aware that words appearing on the label, such as sucrose, glucose, maltose, lactose, corn syrup, or white grape juice concentrate, mean that sugar has been added.
- Look not just at the percentage of calories from fat, but also the number of grams of fat. For every five grams of fat in a serving, you are eating the equivalent of one teaspoon of fat.
- If a snack doesn't provide at least two grams of fiber, it's not a good choice.

DIET ALONE HAS NO EFFECT ON REDUCING INCREASED BLOOD SUGAR VOLATILITY

In a very detailed analysis of the effect of eating a low-glycemic impact diet as demonstrated with the glucose monitoring system (CGMS), recent research that we have been involved with has shown that while levels of blood glucose could be reduced with diet, diet alone did not reduce the tremendous volatility that all of the subjects in the study possessed.

The significance of the results on the effect of a low-glycemic impact diet on blood sugar volatility as shown using the CGMS is quite important. What the results tell us is that because diet did not prevent the peaks and valleys in blood sugar levels, diet alone will fail in stabilizing appetite control in subjects with abdominal obesity.

Increasing Your Intake of Fiber

Increasing your consumption of fiber is central to the success of this program. Eating high fiber foods in abundance reduces hunger and promotes satiety. Fiber also slows the absorption of carbohydrates from food, lowering their glycemic impact. Insoluble fiber such as wheat bran, corn bran, and vegetable fibers increases the volume and viscosity of foods and moderately reduces the glycemic impact of carbohydrates. Soluble fibers such as oat bran, psyllium, and legume fiber, on the other hand, absorb more water and tend to have a greater influence on a food's volume, viscosity, and glycemic impact. Eating an abundance of fiber-rich foods, especially those high in soluble fiber, is central to the success of the Hunger Free Forever program. Here are some suggestions to boost your fiber intake:

- Eat fresh vegetables and fruits for snacks at the first sign of hunger. Eat fruits and vegetables whole, only peeling when necessary.
- Get creative. Add vegetables or fruits to foods (e.g., soups) and modify recipes whenever possible by adding extra fruits or vegetables.
- When you eat grains, try to eat only whole grains. Be sure to read labels to confirm that foods are actually whole grain.
- Use all-bran cereals for breakfast or mixed with plain yogurt as a snack. Add all-bran cereals to other cereals and to other foods whenever possible.
- Boiled whole grains are best. Brown rice, oatmeal, quinoa, couscous, whole barley, barley grits, and barley flakes are good examples. There are many creative ways to prepare boiled grains.
- Try to use legumes as often as possible. Take the time to learn the many ways to use these remarkable foods.

Taking PGX with Every Meal

At the Canadian Center for Functional Medicine, we are credited with the codiscovery of the natural appetite-reducing polysaccharide complex known as PolyGlycopleX (PGX). Working in cooperation with the discoverers of the glycemic index at the University of Toronto, and based upon their initial discoveries, our scientists have developed what is now known to be a completely natural water soluble nonstarch polysaccharide (fiber) complex with greater volume, viscosity, and glycemic index–lowering capabilities of any fiber ever discovered. PGX can be drunk in a glass of water before a meal, sprinkled onto any moist food, taken in capsule form with meals, or consumed as part of a meal replacement beverage. PGX allows you to eat smaller portions of food and still feel full and satisfied for much longer than if you were to consume the food alone. The effect of PGX on appetite and satiety has been demonstrated in double-blind placebo-controlled trials.

One of the remarkable effects of PGX is seen in its impact upon insulin sensitivity and blood sugar control. Double-blind studies have demonstrated that PGX substantially improves insulin sensitivity in insulin-resistant subjects. In a study presented at the American Diabetes Association, a three-week administration of PGX was accompanied by a 50 percent reduction in after-meal insulin levels and a 40 percent improvement in insulin sensitivity along with a highly significant decrease in after-meal blood sugars.

PGX has also been studied at the Glycemic Index Laboratories, whose directors are affiliated with the University of Toronto, where researchers have found that when added to foods or beverages, PGX greatly reduced their glycemic index. The effect of PGX is far superior to that of any other soluble fibers, including beta glucan from oats. This means that any food taken in conjunction with PGX will have a substantially lower glycemic impact.

At the Canadian Center for Functional Medicine, we have demonstrated repeatedly that glycemic volatility is reduced within days by the regular administration of PGX. In most cases, we instruct our patients to begin slowly, starting with 2.5 grams of PGX once per day. We have them gradually increase this over one to two weeks until they are consuming 2.5 to 5 grams of PGX two to three times per day. Most of our heaviest subjects (those over 250 pounds) find that 5 grams of PGX with each meal reduces their appetite substantially. By eliminating their food cravings and choosing healthier foods they achieve remarkable stabilization of their blood sugar levels.

PGX is also available as part of a high-protein meal replacement. One the most successful approaches to weight loss is to consume a PGX-containing meal replacement shake twice per day in place of breakfast and lunch. You are then free to focus on eating one healthy meal per day along with healthy snacks. Additional PGX is usually consumed with your evening meal. This approach is a very simple way to gain the benefits of PGX in terms of stabilization of blood sugar and restoration of insulin sensitivity. After initial weight-loss goals are met, you can begin eating two healthy meals and one meal replacement, all with supplemental PGX, until your weight-loss goals have been achieved. PGX is used as a supplement with the two normal meals. See chapter 10 and appendix D for details about where to obtain PGX and how to use it correctly.

PGX IMPROVES THE METABOLIC SYNDROME

The underlying physiological defect in the metabolic syndrome is insulin resistance and its accompanying elevated insulin levels. PGX has been shown to improve significantly all aspects of the metabolic syndrome. At the annual meeting of the American Diabetes Association in 2004, the results of a clinical study using this proprietary fiber blend were presented by researchers from the Risk Factor Modification Centre at St. Michael's Hospital and the University of Toronto. Subjects with the metabolic syndrome took 3 grams of PGX or a placebo three times a day before meals. After three weeks, there was a 23 percent reduction in after-meal glucose levels, a 40 percent reduction in after-meal insulin release, and a 55.9 percent improvement in whole body insulin sensitivity scores in the group taking PGX. In addition, body fat was reduced by 2.8 percent from baseline over the three-week study period.

Engaging in a Regular Exercise Program: You've Got to Move to Lose

Lack of physical activity promotes insulin resistance. Individuals who are sedentary tend to lose insulin sensitivity even if they don't gain significant amounts of weight. Lack of exercise results in a loss of lean body mass and a reduction in the number and efficiency of insulin receptors in various cells throughout the body. Moderate exercise helps to stabilize the appetite, normalize blood sugar levels, and increase muscle mass, thus increasing your metabolic rate. If you want to get off the blood sugar roller coaster and be free from an appetite in overdrive, you need to make a commitment to regular exercise. (For more information see chapter 7.)

Take a High-Potency Multiple Vitamin and Mineral Formula with Chromium

A deficiency of any one of several key nutrients required for the proper manufacture and function of insulin can lead to impaired sugar metabolism. Especially important are the minerals chromium, magnesium, zinc, and manganese, and B vitamins. The use of a multiple vitamin and mineral supplements is associated with a minimum 30 percent reduction of diabetes risk in men and a 16 percent reduction in risk for women; however, the supplements used in these studies were far from ideal, in our opinion. We believe that by taking a better quality supplement, those reductions can be even greater. In appendix E we provide our recommendations for selecting a high-quality formula.

One of the key nutrients deserves special mention: chromium. Proper blood sugar control requires chromium because it functions in the body as a key constituent of what is referred to as the "glucose tolerance factor." Chromium works closely with insulin in facilitating the uptake of glucose into cells. Without chromium, insulin's action is blocked and glucose levels are elevated. There is evidence that marginal chromium status is quite common in the United States. A chromium deficiency may be an underlying contributing factor to the tremendous number of Americans who have diabetes or hypoglycemia, and are obese.

There have been over twenty clinical studies with chromium supplementation in diabetics. In some of these studies of type 2 diabetes, supplementing the diet with chromium was shown to decrease fasting glucose levels, improve glucose tolerance, lower insulin levels, and decrease total cholesterol and triglyceride levels, while increasing HDL cholesterol levels. Although there are also studies that have not shown chromium to exert much effect in improving glucose tolerance in diabetes, there is no argument that chromium is an important mineral in blood sugar metabolism.

Although there is no RDA for chromium, it appears that we need at least 200mcg each day in our diet. People with diabetes need to supplement 200 to 400mcg per day. Chromium polynicotinate, chromium picolinate, and chromium-enriched yeast are all suitable forms.

TIM'S STORY

I first started gaining weight in my teen years. Up until then I was, by all accounts, a skinny little kid, but in my teens, I developed a laziness that affected all aspects of my life. When it came to eating, because I was a picky eater, my parents basically let me make my own choices. So I tended to choose foods that I thought tasted good, and were fast and easy to make. As is the case with most convenience foods, what I was eating regularly was very high in both calories and fat. The only thing really keeping my weight in check was the variety of sports I was playing throughout the year, but as I entered adulthood, I was playing fewer organized sports, and an athletic 210 pounds became a pudgy 240 pounds.

Every once in a while, I would decide that I needed to lose weight, and would start myself on some sort of exercise program. But because I never bothered to change my eating habits to include a more balanced diet, my laziness would eventually kick in, and my lack of energy would lead me to abandon my well-intended regimen. I knew that I needed to make some serious lifestyle changes if I wanted to be healthier and more energetic, but, sadly, I just couldn't seem to motivate myself to do anything long term if I wasn't seeing immediate results.

A few days after my thirtieth birthday, my wife showed me an ad seeking volunteers for a weight-loss study. She asked me if I would like to check it out with her, so I agreed. I figured I had nothing to lose, but I went thinking this would be yet another failed attempt. It turns out the study involved PGX used in conjunction with a balanced diet and exercise. After having the program explained to us, I thought that it might be something that I could follow without too much hardship, but what really convinced me were some of the issues that surfaced during the medical exam at the beginning of the program. My blood pressure was quite high, and I was showing signs of premature hardening of the arteries. I was only 30 and already going downhill! This was the incentive I needed to start myself down a healthier path. For the first two weeks, my wife and I followed the diet to the letter, using the PGX as directed and working out at the gym. When we went to the first weigh-in at two weeks, I was feeling pretty good and thought that I may have even lost a pound or two in the process. So when I stepped on the scale it took my mind several seconds to grasp the fact that I had lost almost ten pounds in the first two weeks.

After that day, I believe that my life changed forever. I can't imagine returning to the habits that were putting my life in jeopardy, and after losing 45 pounds during the twelve weeks of the program, I know that the lifestyle changes I made with the help of my wife will allow me to maintain a healthy weight for the rest of my life. I have never felt better than I do today, and I have PGX products to thank for helping me to finally conquer the laziness that had threatened my health for far too long.

Tim, age 30

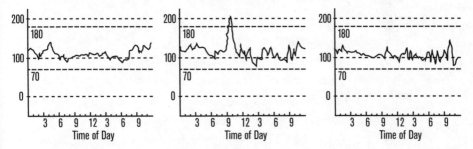

Figure 3.7. Tim's Continuous Blood Glucose Before Starting the Hunger Free Forever Program.

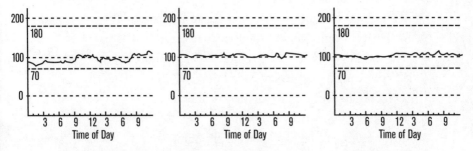

Figure 3.8. Tim's Continuous Blood Glucose 6 Weeks After Starting the Hunger Free Forever Program.

CHAPTER SUMMARY

- Blood sugar volatility is a major factor for the increased appetite and frequent food cravings so typical of individuals who are struggling with their weight.
- Reducing blood sugar volatility is accomplished by following dietary, lifestyle, and supplement strategies that improve the sensitivity of cells throughout the body to insulin.
- Low-carb and no-carb diets can produce quick and dramatic results, but they most often lead to rebound weight gain.
- The body works hard to keep blood sugar normal as insulin resistance develops by releasing higher than normal amounts of insulin.
- We commonly discover fasting insulin levels to be two to three times the normal value even in many who are only modestly overweight.
- Insulin is an anabolic hormone that promotes the growth of fat cells.
- Unless insulin sensitivity is restored, weight loss through dieting is an uphill battle at best and is impossible for most people.
- The brain can become insulin resistant along with the rest of the body. This insulin resistance plays an important role in the loss of after-meal satiety that accompanies weight gain.
- Although we know that the control of appetite is influenced by a whole orchestra of hormones, peptides, and neurotransmitters, glucose can still be considered as a lead player and perhaps the conductor of this orchestra.
- Rapid and deep drops in blood sugar are particularly associated with very strong—and in some cases irresistible—urges to eat.
- The five key steps to reduce blood sugar volatility involve:
  1. Following a low glycemic load diet.
  2. Increasing your intake of dietary fiber.
  3. Taking PGX with every meal.
  4. Engaging in a regular exercise program.
  5. Taking a high potency multiple vitamin with chromium.
- Two tools to help you choose carbohydrates wisely and to con-

sume modest portion sizes are the glycemic index (GI) and glycemic load (GL).

- If you want to get off the blood sugar roller coaster and be free from an appetite in overdrive, you need to make a commitment to regular exercise.
- Blood sugar control requires chromium because it functions in the body as a key constituent of the glucose tolerance factor.

4

DEVELOP EATING STRATEGIES
FOR HIGH SATIETY

Rather than focusing on a complex diet with numerous rules, we have found great success at our center in helping people use principles and strategies that allow them to improve blood sugar control, tame their appetite, and experience a high level of satiety even when eating lower calorie portions of food. By focusing on eating strategies rather than a specific diet, our program becomes an acceptable, long-term way of life rather than something that you endure for a few weeks and then forget as you migrate back to your old habits once again. Instead, once you have your appetite under control with the Hunger Free Forever program, you can make other sensible changes in your lifestyle habits and behaviors to help you gain healthy control over your weight as a way of life.

Appetite reflects a very complex system that has evolved to help humans deal with food shortages. As a result, it is extremely biased toward weight gain. It makes sense that people who survived famines were those who were more adept at storing fat than burning it. So there is a built-in tendency for all of us to overeat even though in developed countries food is readily available.

The flip side of an increased appetite is the feeling of satiety. We feel that the most exciting area in obesity research is the science of satiety—the study of what properties, nutrients, or elements in food result in a sense of fullness or satiety. There are several important properties of food that can either promote satiety or contribute to overconsumption. Choosing foods that promote satiety and avoiding or limiting the intake of those foods that contribute to overconsumption is critical to long-term weight control.

Ultimately the satiety-promoting effects of a food relate to its influence on the appetite control centers in the brain. In addition to blood glucose fluctuations and mechanical effects occurring in the stomach and gastrointestinal tract, there are a number of hunger and satiety chemicals secreted by the pancreas, intestinal cells, and fat cells that play a huge role in regulating appetite. We will discuss some of these important regulators below as well as the three most important properties that determine a food's ability to create a significant and sustainable sense of satiety. They are:

- Glycemic impact (the impact of a food on your blood sugar)
- Volume (how much space a food occupies in your stomach)
- Viscosity (the thickness of a food as it passes through your digestive tract)

Since we discussed the role of glycemic impact in chapter 3, we will focus on the importance of volume and viscosity in this chapter.

THE INFLUENCE OF FOOD VOLUME ON SATIETY

Most foods in the modern Western diet are packed with calories for the amount of volume they occupy in the stomach. This means you will have a tendency to eat far too many calories before your stomach feels at all full. For example, a Wendy's Classic double with cheese and a large order of fries occupies about two cups of volume in your stomach, but contributes about 1,300 calories to your diet. Since the stomach of an obese person can hold up to four quarts of volume, the two cups of burger and fries wouldn't necessarily create a great sense of fullness even though the calorie intake is over the top. In contrast, two cups of chopped apple contains only 120 calories! In other words, you would have to eat twenty-two cups of chopped apple to consume the same number of calories as just one burger and an order of fries. Even a huge eater would probably find it impossible to eat 1,300 calories of apple because this would take up about five and a half quarts of volume in their stomach—they might explode before they got it all down.

In addition to being low in volume for the amount of calories they contain, typical foods in the Western diet are also very low in thickness or viscosity. They become thin watery liquids once they are chewed, swallowed, and mixed with fluids and acid in the stomach. Low-viscosity foods move through the digestive tract very quickly and are rapidly absorbed, which means that your digestive system will be looking for more food shortly after you've eaten your meal. As well, many of the foods typical of the modern Western diet contain highly refined carbohydrates, which tend to result in a rapid and excessive elevation of after-meal blood sugars (high glycemic impact). Foods that cause blood sugar to surge rapidly after meals may contribute to initial satiety, but they backfire and end up actually promoting excessive food intake in the hours that follow.

Fast foods, junk foods, and sugary drinks are the worst kind of foods to eat if you want to achieve a sense of fullness or satiety while reducing your caloric intake. The same applies to many foods that are made with refined flour or added sugar, and to most high-fat foods. These sorts of foods taste sumptuous and are loaded with calories. Because of this, you tend to eat so quickly that you've overeaten before you even feel full. Sit down to your typical steak and potatoes, pasta, pizza, fried chicken, or burger and fries when you are really hungry and you can easily eat three or four times your caloric requirement for that meal before you even feel a sense of satiety. In terms of calories, it takes an enormous quantity of those foods to fill your stomach, and because they become low-viscosity liquids once chewed and diluted with stomach juices, they pass through the digestive tract very rapidly, making you feel ready for more food a short time later.

How Does Volume Affect Satiety?

The volume of food consumed may affect satiety in several ways. First, a larger volume of food can affect the perception of how much food is being consumed. Next, more time is required to consume foods that are larger in volume than those that are smaller in volume. This effect

THE SATIETY EFFECT OF AIR

One of the leading proponents of reducing caloric intake by volumetric eating is Barbara Rolls, Ph.D., professor of nutrition and director of the Laboratory for the Study of Human Ingestive Behavior at Pennsylvania State University. Dr. Rolls has authored over 200 research articles, most relating to the concept that people feel full because of the amount of food they eat, not because of the number of calories or the grams of fat, protein, or carbohydrates consumed.

One of our favorite research studies conducted by Dr. Rolls demonstrates the fact that you can increase the volume of food without increasing the amount of calories and still promote satiety. Dr. Rolls and colleagues enrolled twenty-eight lean men into the study and had them consume breakfast, lunch, and dinner in the laboratory one day per week for four weeks. Over the course of the trial they consumed a milkshake that varied in volume (300, 450, and 600 ml), but not in calories, as a "preload" thirty minutes before lunch to compare the effect on satiety compared to the first day in the laboratory when no preload was served. The difference in volume in the milkshakes was the result of different amounts of air pumped into the milkshakes; otherwise they were identical.

The results indicated that the volume of the milkshake significantly affected calorie consumption at lunch. When given the 600ml preload, there was a 12 percent reduced calorie intake at lunch (400 fewer calories) compared to the 300ml group. Subjects also reported greater reductions in hunger and greater increases in fullness after consumption of both the 450 and 600ml preloads than after the 300ml preload.

In our practice, we have found that air-filled foods can be very filling. A great example is the blender smoothie made with the meal replacement formulas containing PGX and whey protein. The whey protein foams when vigorously blended. This effect nearly doubles the volume of the smoothie, giving you a lot of fullness with few calories, and it tastes great as well.

could be substantial in that it allows the necessary time for important feedback mechanisms associated with satiety to reach the appetite control centers in the brain.

Perhaps the biggest impact of increased food volume as it leads to reduced caloric intake relates to its effect on producing distension of the stomach. In fact, the air in Dr. Rolls's milkshakes (see "The Satiety Effect of Air," page 67) produced greater distension of the stomach and therefore influenced subjective responses related to hunger and appetite. In both animal and human studies, the degree of gastric distension is known to affect food intake, particularly by effecting the feeling that you have had enough.

In addition to creating a sense of fullness, the volume of a food influences satiety by slowing down gastric (stomach) emptying. In essence, the longer the food stays in the stomach, the stronger and longer lasting is the satiety feedback to the appetite control centers of the brain.

Taking Advantage of High-Volume and High-Viscosity Foods

To promote a high level of satiety, you must incorporate a variety of foods in your diet each day that are lower in calories but high in volume, high in viscosity, and low in their glycemic impact. Particularly, if you eat these kinds of foods at the beginning of most meals, your initial hunger will begin to diminish and when you turn to the parts of your meal that are higher in calories, you will be able to eat slower and feel satisfied with a smaller portion size. For example, if you start a meal by eating a very large salad with a minimal amount of low-calorie dressing, or a large bowl of low-calorie, high-fiber soup, you will start to feel full before you turn to the higher calorie foods of your meal like steak and potato, and you will be able to savor smaller portions without being tempted to overeat.

Foods like meat, bread, and pasta can all be an important part of a healthy diet, but they are low in volume and high in calories and need to be eaten in moderation to avoid weight gain. By taming your appetite with foods that are higher in volume and viscosity early in your meal, you give your stomach a chance to communicate to the brain that you are starting to feel satisfied before you turn to the higher calorie foods in your meal. Thus, when you get to those foods, you can practice eating slowly and savoring every bite, while being careful to eat smaller portions and avoid going back for seconds. With this strategy, even very big eaters can push away from the dinner table feeling full without overeating in terms of calories. There is nothing wrong with having a full stomach as long as the calories in your stomach are low enough to promote weight loss.

Learning to incorporate high-volume and -viscosity foods into each meal and learning to choose volumetric snacks over calorie-packed snacks and beverages can have a very significant impact on satiety. As well, learning simple ways to increase the volumetric properties of recipes and even how to make volumetric choices when eating out can both be used as simple strategies to feel full after every meal and still reduce your caloric intake significantly. For those who master these principles, weight loss can be hunger free and enjoyable, even when their weight goal takes many months to achieve. That's because this is not just another diet. It is an enjoyable way of life!

PGX AND THE SCIENCE OF SATIETY

Our appetite is extremely biased toward weight gain. Nonetheless, satiety can be achieved in a manner that tilts in favor of weight loss. Your greatest ally in this battle is PGX. This complex of natural supersoluble nonstarch polysaccharides (fiber) exerts a powerful effect on promoting satiety via several mechanisms. PGX absorbs several hundred times its weight in water, thus adding substantially to the volume of your meal without adding any additional calories. The volumetric effects of PGX result in a sense of fullness soon after it is consumed. In fact, when mixed with water, it becomes the most viscous dietary fiber ever developed. This means that PGX mixes with food in the stomach, increasing its thickness or viscosity, slowing gastric emptying, and then prolonging the digestion and absorption of any food. By slowing gastric emptying and digestion, PGX promotes a prolonged sense of satiety. It also greatly slows the absorption of carbohydrates, lowering the glycemic impact of these foods. Research at the University of Toronto also suggests that PGX increases the level of important appetite-reducing peptides and hormones such as GLP-1 (see box below) and cholecystokinin (CCK). All in all, if you take PGX with each meal, you will be able to eat less and feel more satisfied. All of our weight-loss patients use PGX as a central part of their high satiety eating strategy.

GLP-1, L-CELLS, AND PGX

An emerging mechanism further explaining the effects of PGX on satiety and blood sugar control involves a hormone secreted in the small intestine and colon known as glucagon-like peptide-1 (GLP-1). This important hormone is secreted by L-cells in the small intestine and colon in response to food intake. GLP-1 exerts multiple effects as it has been shown to:

• Improve blood sugar control
• Promote satiety, leading to reduction of food intake
• Regulate the rate of gastric emptying, thereby reducing after-meal glucose levels

A synthetic form of GLP-1 is an approved drug in the treatment of type 2 diabetes, but, like insulin, it must be injected twice daily. The drug, called Byetta (exenatide), often produces significant weight loss as it makes most feel full, leading to reduced food intake.

PGX has been shown to raise GLP-1 levels naturally and does not have to be administered by injection. We believe this effect is two-fold. First, the release of GLP-1 is in direct response to PGX. Second, the PGX may increase the number of L-cells that produce GLP-1 in the small intestine and colon.

What appears to make PGX more effective than other fiber sources may be that it leads to pulses of GLP-1 release into the bloodstream as it passes throughout the entire digestive tract. Since naturally produced GLP-1 is broken down by the body within two minutes after it is formed, repeated pulses of release would be necessary to produce a prolonged effect. The prolonged effect of PGX on satiety would support this mechanism.

THE WEIGHT-LOSS EQUATION

In order to lose one pound of fat by diet alone in one week, an individual needs to have a negative calorie intake of 500 calories per day or 3,500 calories per week, since there are 3,500 calories in one pound of fat. To lose two pounds of fat each week, there must be a negative caloric balance of 1,000 calories a day. To reduce one's caloric intake by 1,000 calories per day is often difficult and can even backfire. If you cut calories too severely, which for most people can occur when daily caloric intake is less than 1,000 calories per day, much of the weight you lose will be muscle. One pound of fat contains 3,500 calories, but one pound of muscle has only 600 calories. This means that during severe or very imbalanced diets, you can lose muscle very quickly because you have to burn almost six times as many calories to burn off a pound of fat than if you are burning muscle for calories.

To increase one's caloric output by burning an additional 1,000 calories per day by exercise, a person would need to jog for 90 minutes, play tennis for 2 hours, or take a brisk two and a half hour walk. As well, although moderate exercise tends to help normalize appetite, severe exercise can provoke a profound increase in appetite and can even promote binge eating in some people.

The most sensible approach to weight loss is to decrease caloric intake and increase moderate exercise simultaneously. Reading labels and paying close attention to the caloric content of foods can be very valuable. As well, making frequent use of Internet resources such as the USDA's National Nutrient Database (www.nal.usda.gov/fnic/food comp/search/) or private nutrition services such as www.calorieking .com/foods or www.nutritiondata.com can help you develop even more calorie awareness. Consulting with a registered dietician can also be an invaluable way to become more intelligent about your food choices for weight loss.

Calories Do Count

All calories come from fat, protein, or carbohydrate. There is nothing higher in calories than fat. Pure fat or oil (oil is just liquid fat) contains 9 calories per gram. On the other hand, carbohydrates (starch or sugar)

HOW CAN A DIETITIAN HELP YOU LOSE WEIGHT?

Registered dietitians (R.D.s) are acknowledged professionals uniquely trained to advise you on diet, food, and nutrition. They can separate fact from fiction and healthy eating plans from unsafe diets, and translate the science of nutrition into healthy food choices. They can help you become more aware of your eating behaviors, and they can help you to understand where the extra calories have come from that have resulted in your weight gain.

Dietitians are experts on providing practical information about how to change your individual diet into a healthier lifestyle. Dietitians give client-centered care, so whether you don't know where to begin or are well versed in nutrition and just need a hand, they are able to assess your needs and get you on the road to manageable weight loss and improved health and wellness.

To find a registered dietician in your area go to the Web sites of the American Dietetic Association, (eatright.org) or Dietitians of Canada, (www.dietitians.ca).

and protein contain 4 calories per gram. Although fat indeed contains the most calories for its weight or volume, if you overeat calories from foods high in protein or carbohydrate it is still easy to gain weight. The low-fat food craze was followed by the low-carbohydrate food craze— and society has gotten fatter with each passing fad. The reality is that if you eat too much of any calorie-containing food, you will gain weight.

Everyone hates to count calories, but unfortunately, calories do count when it comes to your weight. Calories are a measurement of the amount of energy stored inside a given food or beverage. If you consume more calories than your body burns, you will gain weight. There is no magic pill, magic diet, or even magic workout that will let you eat more calories than you burn without those excessive calories turning into fat. You can do several things to increase the amount of calories your body burns and we will address these in chapter 8. However, by far the most important thing that we can help you to do is learn how to eat fewer calories than your body needs while avoiding hunger and experiencing satiety with every meal.

Moderation Is Essential with High Caloric–Density Foods

Becoming aware of where extra and unnecessary calories are coming from is essential if you want to get your weight under control. One of the most important things that we teach our weight-loss patients is the concept of caloric density. Caloric density refers to the amount of calories contained in a given weight and volume of food. Foods that are high in caloric density are foods that pack on the calories in a very small weight and volume. For example, a cup of peanuts contains nearly 1,000 calories (a very high caloric–density food) whereas a cup of chopped apple contains only 60 calories (a very low caloric–density food). This doesn't mean that you should never eat peanuts and only eat apples. It does mean that you can easily eat enough nuts in a few minutes to pack on the weight if you eat those nuts mindlessly. Our weight-loss patients are actually all encouraged to eat nuts, but only in appropriate portion sizes: a small handful or no more than one-quarter cup of raw or lightly dry roasted, unsalted nuts per day. In modest amounts, nuts have been shown to help in weight loss as a result of their ability to promote satiety and improve insulin sensitivity. However, even with healthy high-calorie foods like nuts, the saying "everything in moderation" truly applies.

Certainly there are many nutritious foods that we need to eat for good health, and foods that we might not want to live without that have a very high-caloric density (can you say chocolate?). The key to being able to consume these foods regularly without gaining weight primarily depends on first eating substantial amounts of low caloric–density, volumetric foods to reduce appetite and consistently promote satiety. In this way, you will be able to maintain careful portion control when eating high caloric–density foods and not have to depend on willpower when your appetite is in overdrive.

For example, some of our most successful weight-loss participants have learned to limit themselves to a tiny square of chocolate two or three times per week rather than avoid it altogether. They have learned to reward themselves for losing weight by savoring a small bit of chocolate (the size of a thumbprint) as slowly as they can eat it. If you take tiny nibbles and let it melt slowly in your mouth, it can be a real treat. After this chocolate experience is over, all you have is the memory of it anyway, and the enjoyment of this little bit of chocolate is almost as great as if you were to eat a few hundred calories of chocolate.

Fiber, Water, and Caloric Density

Fiber and water are the two most important ingredients in food that can add volume and viscosity without contributing calories. It has been well recognized for many years that eating high-fiber foods contributes to weight loss. Fiber refers to carbohydrates that cannot be digested; they contribute very few calories to the diet. Fiber can be insoluble (it doesn't absorb much water) or soluble (the fiber absorbs water like a sponge). High-fiber foods help you to feel full on fewer calories than low-fiber foods. Fiber also mixes with food, creating viscosity and slowing digestion, thus contributing to prolonged satiety and reducing after-meal blood sugar surges.

The most important foods for promoting satiety are those which are very high in fiber and contain a great deal of water. Low-fat salads, high-fiber soups, legumes, raw or cooked nonstarchy vegetables, boiled whole grains like brown rice or oatmeal, and low-fat stews are all foods that must become a major part of your lifestyle if you want to lose weight and keep it off for good. Our most successful weight-loss participants have made the effort to find a wide variety of ways to incorporate these kinds of foods into their daily life. We will provide you with a wealth of recipes in chapter 11 to make high-fiber, volumetric foods a delicious part of your diet.

In addition to consuming more high-fiber, volumetric foods, all of our weight-loss participants add PGX fiber to their meals two to three times per day. PGX has the highest volume and viscosity of any fiber. A dosage of 2.5 to 5 grams of PGX can be added to water and taken before meals, added to soups, yogurt, or any moist food, taken in capsule form or consumed as part of a high-protein meal replacement beverage. Because PGX absorbs hundreds of times its weight in water, it begins to act very quickly in the stomach to create a sense of fullness.

This allows you to eat smaller food portions and still experience satiety. Because PGX continues to maintain its viscosity throughout the digestive tract, it slows digestion and greatly reduces blood sugar surges while promoting a prolonged sense of satiety. If used in conjunction with high-fiber, volumetric foods, the appetite-reducing qualities of those foods are substantially magnified and weight loss becomes significantly easier than with volumetric eating alone.

The Importance of Water

People who want to lose weight need to ensure that they are drinking adequate amounts of water or other low- or no-calorie beverages. In many cases, a hunger pang can be relieved by simply drinking a glass of water. Why? It may be because mild dehydration created a sensation that is perceived as hunger. It may also be because water added volume to the stomach. However, since water and most other beverages are quickly absorbed, they reduce hunger only briefly and have no prolonged impact on satiety. Those who are successful in losing weight and keeping it off have learned to drink plenty of water or other noncaloric beverages, but they also consume significant amounts of water in the form of low-fat, high-fiber soups, vegetables, fruits, boiled whole grains, and other volumetric foods. The fiber in these foods holds on to the water and makes these foods more volumetric.

BEWARE OF SWEETENED DRINKS

Sugary drinks like soda pop, sweetened iced tea, and fruit juice are probably the worst ways to provide your body with calories if you want to lose weight. These high caloric–density beverages are absorbed very rapidly into the blood, so they contribute minimally to a sense of fullness but result in a rapid surge of blood sugar accompanied by a significant release of insulin. Even in nondiabetics, sugary drinks contribute to a significant increase in appetite in the hours that follow. Other than the occasional small servings of pure high-

(continued on next page)

antioxidant fruit juice, we urge that you completely avoid all sugary drinks.

Learning to stay well hydrated with water, sparkling mineral water, unsweetened tea, low-calorie broths, and other healthy, non-caloric beverages is an important habit to develop if you want to maintain an ideal weight for life. Although diet sodas contain no cal-ories, they contain numerous unhealthy chemicals and keep your taste buds and brain attuned to desiring very sweet flavors. Diet sodas are certainly better than sugar-laden beverages, but you're far better off to develop a taste for water, mineral water, and healthy, un-sweetened teas.

Choose Lower Caloric-Density Foods

All foods are composed of some combination of fat, carbohydrate, pro-tein, fiber, and water. Foods that are highest in fat tend to be those with the highest caloric density, followed by those that are high-carbohydrate or high-protein, unless they are also high in water and fiber. Foods that are high in water and fiber have the lowest caloric density. For exam-ple, vegetables and fresh fruit are high in water and fiber.

Salads with minimal or low-calorie dressings; roasted or grilled vegetables; hearty vegetable or legume-based soups; boiled whole grains; legume dishes; high-protein, low-calorie smoothies; and fresh, nontropical fruits are all examples of foods that can be enjoyed liber-ally because they promote satiety while adding abundant nutrients and minimal calories. The key to keeping these foods high in volume and yet low in their caloric density is to avoid adding more than a small amount of fat or other high-calorie embellishments. Although our taste buds have become accustomed to high-fat dressings, vegetables drowned in rich dressings or high-fat sauces are high-calorie land-mines being added to otherwise low-calorie, high-volume foods. Chapter 11 provides recipes and reveals the secrets to making low caloric–density, volumetric foods taste fantastic.

IT TAKES TIME TO KNOW YOU HAVE HAD ENOUGH

Your body does possess some mechanisms to sense the number of calories that you consume, but it takes quite a while for this information
to reach the brain because your body really doesn't know how many
calories you've consumed until the food you've eaten is digested and
fully absorbed. This is why, for example, it is so easy to overeat fast
food. You can easily eat 2,000 calories of fast food in a few minutes and
not even realize that you've eaten three times your caloric requirements
for that meal until an hour or two after the meal is over. On the opposite end of the spectrum, if you take the time at the beginning of your
meal to eat a large salad with minimal dressing (we tell our patients to
have the dressing on the side and dip their fork into the dressing each
time before they pick up the vegetables), by the time you finish the
salad, your appetite has diminished considerably and you will find it
easy to eat small portions of the higher caloric density foods in your
meal.

You might be accustomed to eating, for example, a large baked
potato with all the fixings, a 12-ounce steak, small salad, and a piece of
pie for dessert. Instead, you could start the meal with a really big salad
and a small amount of dressing or a large bowl of low-fat, high-fiber
soup. Then you could slowly eat a 4-ounce piece of lean steak and a
small baked potato perhaps with plain yogurt, a few bacon bits, some
chives, a bit of sea salt, and a teaspoon of flaxseed oil. The salad or
high-fiber soup takes quite a while to eat and it gives your stomach
time to tell your brain that you don't have to eat that much more
food. Researchers at Pennsylvania State University found that when
subjects consumed a high-volume, low-calorie soup before a meal, it
led to a 20 percent reduction in total calories consumed for the meal.
When you're not so hungry, you will find that you can easily slow down
and savor every bite, rather than just wolfing your food down. For dessert, you can have something as simple as an apple or a bowl of raspberries later on if you start to feel a bit hungry. In the end, you will
be able to finish your dinners feeling more satisfied, but with half the
calories.

Never Eat When You Are Too Hungry

If you're like most of us, your mother probably always warned you not to eat before your meals lest you spoil your appetite. At our center, we teach people something quite contrary. In reality, your worst enemy is excessive hunger and you need to avoid, at all costs, sitting down to a meal when you are more than just mildly hungry. Many of our overweight patients have great discipline over their eating habits for part of the day. Many skip breakfast and eat a very light lunch, but their real eating begins when they get home. The majority of overweight people really seem to enjoy diving into their evening meal when they are as hungry as a bear coming out of hibernation. They tend to gobble down their food, often having seconds or even thirds followed by desserts, and then nibbling throughout the evening.

Instead, we stress the importance of spreading your calories throughout the day. First and foremost, you must learn to have a good breakfast with adequate protein and fiber. You must also have a healthy lunch and should always have a small snack between each meal. Most important, you will need to learn to "spoil your appetite" before dinner. Rather than sitting down to eat when you are overly hungry, we encourage you to eat a low calorie–density snack to calm down your appetite before your evening meal. An apple with six to ten almonds, a serving of plain yogurt with bran cereal, a handful of baby carrots with a couple tablespoons of seeds, or a hard-boiled egg and a couple pieces of celery are just a few of things that can be eaten thirty minutes to one hour before the evening meal to help reduce hunger and make it less likely that you will end up overeating. As well, most of our patients find it helpful to add 2.5 to 5 grams of PGX to a glass of water or 3 to 6 PGX Softgel capsules fifteen to twenty minutes before each meal.

FAT, PROTEIN, AND SATIETY

Although we have focused upon the importance of glycemic impact, food volume, and viscosity in the promotion and maintenance of satiety, there are other important factors that must be considered if you want to experience effective weight loss, free from the discomfort of excessive hunger. Both fat and protein contribute to a food's taste as well as its ability to initiate and maintain satiety. Meals that are high in volume and viscosity but lack protein and fat are less effective in eliminating hunger and creating a prolonged sense of satisfaction.

Even though fat is so high in calories, it is critical to consume adequate amounts of healthy fats if you want to lose weight. The biggest mistake is simply eating too much fat, and thus, too many calories. All it takes is a very small amount of fat to promote satiety. As little as 2 grams of fat in a stomach full of food will significantly add to the satiety-inducing effects of that food. There are also numerous other health benefits of certain types of fat. Olive oil, avocado, nuts and seeds, fatty fish, fish oils, and coconut oil are just a few examples of fats that should be consumed regularly for health and satiety. The key to gaining the benefits of these healthy fats is real moderation. All fats contain about 9 calories per gram so none of them should be used liberally. Books promoting fats for weight loss suggest that you can eat any quantity of certain kinds of oils and still lose weight. That's pure foolishness. Striking a balance between the low-fat craze and overzealous use of healthy oils is the key to finding their true benefits.

Good Fats Versus Bad Fats

One of the key determinants of whether a fat is good or bad is its effect on cellular membranes and, as a result, the action of insulin. Membranes are made mostly of fatty acids. What determines the type of fatty acid present in the cell membrane is the type of fat you consume. A diet composed mostly of saturated fat, animal fatty acids, and trans fatty acids (from margarine, shortening, and other sources of hydrogenated vegetable oils), and high in cholesterol, results in membranes that are much less fluid in nature than the membranes in a person who consumes optimum levels of unsaturated fatty acids. Without a healthy membrane, cells lose their ability to hold water, vital nutrients, and electrolytes. They also lose their ability to communicate with other cells and be controlled by regulating hormones including insulin. Without the right type of fats in cell membranes, cells simply do not function properly. Considerable evidence indicates that cell membrane dysfunction is a critical factor in the development of insulin resistance, obesity, and diabetes. So it is critical to effective long-term weight management that you eat the right types of fats.

The type of dietary fat profile linked to insulin resistance is an abundance of saturated fat and trans fatty acids along with a relative insufficiency of monounsaturated and omega-3 fatty acids. This means that in order to improve insulin action, we should reduce our intake of saturated fats by eating leaner cuts of meat and choosing nonfat dairy options, as well as eliminating trans fatty acids from our diet and focusing instead on monounsaturated fatty acids and omega-3 fatty acids. The best sources of monounsaturated fats are olive oil, nuts, nut oils, and canola oil. Although monounsaturated fats are not as unsaturated as polyunsaturated, they still contribute to healthier cell membranes because they are more fluid than saturated fats. And, because they only have one unsaturated bond, they are more stable and provide better protection against oxidative damage to cell membranes than polyunsaturated oils.

While olive oil and canola oil are by far the most popular monounsaturated fats in use, macadamia nut oil is superior to cook with because of lower levels of polyunsaturated oil (3 percent for macadamia nut oil versus 8 percent for olive and 23 percent for canola). As a result, while olive oil and canola oil can form lipid peroxides (rancid byproducts created through oxidation) at relatively low cooking temperatures, macadamia nut oil is stable at much higher temperatures (over twice that of olive oil and four times more stable than canola). Macadamia oil, like olive oil is also very high in natural antioxidants. In fact it contains over 4.5 times the amount of vitamin E as olive oil. For more information on macadamia nut oil, visit www.mac nutoil.com.

Another important aspect to getting the right type of oils in your diet is to eat fish rich in the omega-3 fatty acids, such as salmon, mackerel, herring, and halibut. While we are encouraging you to eat more fish, we need to give you some guidelines. Nearly all fish contain trace amounts of methyl mercury. In most cases, this is of little concern because the level is so low. The fish most likely to have the lowest level of methyl mercury are salmon (usually undetectable levels), cod, mackerel, cold-water tuna, farm-raised catfish, and herring. Certain seafood, particularly swordfish, shark, and some other large predatory fish, may contain high levels of methyl mercury. Choose from the low-mercury group and limit your intake to no more than four servings per week maximum.

Adding a high-quality fish oil supplement free of the mercury, PCBs, dioxins, and other contaminants often found in fish to your daily routine provides extra insurance that you are getting sufficient levels of omega-3 fatty acids. Take enough of the supplement to provide 1,000mg daily of the key omega-3 fatty acids EPA and DHA.

Protein

Protein, too, has been well demonstrated to be vital in the maintenance of healthy appetite control. It is particularly important to start the day with a high-protein breakfast, but protein needs to be eaten throughout the day to avoid excess hunger and to promote prolonged satiety. Eggs or egg whites with grilled vegetables, grilled chicken with vegetables, yogurt and bran cereal, scrambled tofu with vegetables, or high-protein volumetric meal replacement drinks or smoothies are all excellent items to consider as part of a satiety-promoting breakfast. Whey protein is one of nature's highest quality proteins and is a very useful (perhaps essential) ingredient that can be used easily to increase the protein content of any meal. Whey protein has also been shown to promote satiety. Smoothies made with whey protein or meal replacement shakes that contain whey protein and PGX are excellent high-satiety breakfast foods.

It is also very important to include protein in your other meals. Protein sources should be very lean and can include lean meats and poultry, fish, low-fat dairy products, eggs or egg whites, legumes, or tofu. The body looks for protein and the appetite will increase if you deprive the body of adequate amounts of this important nutrient group. Protein also supports the growth of muscle, helps to stabilize blood sugar, and provides prolonged energy. However, it is often hard to consume protein without also consuming an excessive amount of fat so be sure to choose only lean protein foods.

We always instruct our patients to focus on eating volumetric, low caloric–density foods as the main part of their meal and then carefully and slowly consume smaller portions of higher caloric-density foods such as meats. Some higher protein foods are very hard to find in low-fat varieties. For example, cheese is a favorite food for many overweight people. Even though cheese is high in protein, it is usually loaded with fat and is one of the highest caloric-density foods in existence. If you want to lose weight and still eat cheese, you must keep your portion sizes very small. For higher fat versions of cheese, limit your daily cheese intake to a portion the size of your thumb. Yogurt cheeses and ricotta are examples of low-fat alternates to higher fat cheeses that can be eaten in larger portions. You can find recommendations for incorporating healthy sources of protein into your diet in chapter 10.

One of the best sources of protein for weight loss is legumes as they are rich not only in protein but also insoluble fiber, thereby increasing satiety as well as exerting a number of other beneficial effects. Learning to cook with a variety of beans, lentils, split peas, and legume products such as tofu can be one of the most valuable skills that you can learn. When you really become familiar with the hundreds of ways you can use these inexpensive and healthy foods, you will have discovered one of the best ways to fall in love with the high-satiety way of life. Buying these ingredients in bulk, cooking them in batches with a pressure cooker or slowly on the stove top will allow you to freeze several single-recipe portions that can then be taken out to prepare quick and easy meals. We provide you with numerous cooking hints and recipes to take advantage of these fantastic foods in chapter 10.

CHAPTER SUMMARY

- Once you have your appetite under control with the Hunger Free Forever program, you can make other sensible changes in their lifestyle, habits, and behaviors that will help you gain healthy control over your weight as a way of life.
- Appetite reflects a very complex system that has evolved to help humans deal with food shortages.

- The three most important properties that determine a food's ability to create a significant and sustainable sense of satiety are:
  - Glycemic impact (the impact of a food on your blood sugar)
  - Volume (how much space a food occupies in your stomach)
  - Viscosity (the thickness of a food as it passes through your digestive tract)
- The volume of a food fills your stomach and makes you feel full; the viscosity of a food slows digestion and keeps you feeling full; the glycemic impact of a food determines if it will result in a blood sugar surge and if it does, it will promote food cravings and overeating later.
- Becoming aware of where extra and unnecessary calories are coming from is essential if you want to get your weight under control.
- Fiber and water are the two most important ingredients in food that can add volume and viscosity without contributing calories.
- Eat higher amounts of foods with a lower caloric density.
- Eating regular meals is important to prevent excessive hunger, which can sabotage your weight-loss program.
- PGX possesses an ability to increase insulin sensitivity, reduce blood sugar volatility, and produce volumetric effects. It is very viscous and produces a targeted effect of reducing those factors that increase appetite while simultaneously increasing those factors that decrease appetite.
- Both protein and fat contribute to a food's taste as well as its ability to initiate and maintain satiety.
- Meals that are high in volume and viscosity, but lack protein and fat, are less effective in eliminating hunger and creating a prolonged sense of satisfaction.
- Moderation is the key when consuming high caloric–density foods.
- Whey protein is one of nature's highest quality proteins and can be used easily to increase the protein content of any meal.
- Whey protein promotes satiety.

5

TRANSFORM YOUR HABITS, TRANSFORM YOUR LIFE

We are all creatures of habit. We all tend to repeat behaviors that relieve discomfort and make us feel good until those behaviors evolve into habits that form a real grip on us. In many ways, our habits define who we are and what we will become. Most people with weight problems know that they have to change their eating habits, but they are fearful of losing the comfort and pleasure that food provides. Popular diets are appealing because they promise short-term solutions, but in reality, they don't address the real reasons why we are overweight—our eating habits.

Most people can occasionally muster up the courage to lose some weight through dieting. However, because diets don't reduce our appetite or help us change and improve our eating habits, we eventually gravitate back to our old habits again. The kind of food we eat, when we eat, and how fast and how much we eat are all choices and behaviors that need to be aligned with our weight-loss goals if we want to achieve long-term success.

What our patients tell us over and over again is that the Hunger Free Forever program has finally given them the power that diets never could. They all knew that to lose weight they needed to make wiser food choices, eat less, and exercise, but willpower alone was not enough. The Hunger Free Forever program freed them from an appetite in overdrive and gave them new energy so that they could make long-term changes in their eating and exercise habits without the discomfort and temptation they had always experienced with diets alone.

TRANSFORM YOUR HABITS, TRANSFORM YOUR LIFE

At our clinical research center, we consider restoring normal appetite control to be central to the success of our program. The first step, taming the appetite, involves helping you to enrich your diet with foods that are high in volume and viscosity, and low in their glycemic impact. We also make extensive use of the supersoluble fiber, PGX. In addition to bringing about a sense of fullness, this simple program dramatically stabilizes blood sugar control, getting you off the blood sugar roller coaster. At that point, appetite diminishes significantly and unhealthy food cravings are dramatically decreased or eliminated. Early in the program you will likely experience an improvement in your sleep and energy levels and notice that your belly begins to decrease in size even before your weight goes down on the scale.

In order to experience these positive changes, you must adopt the following five key habits:

1) Tailor your food portions.
2) Take your time when eating.
3) Think ahead and plan what you are going to eat.
4) Turn to delicious, healthy foods and turn away from problem foods.
5) Take time to cultivate healthy habits and terminate bad habits and food addictions.

Are You Ready for Change?

The primary factor that will determine whether you are successful at losing weight and whether that success will last is how ready you are for change. Behavioral scientists have determined five stages of change necessary to overcome bad habits, lifestyle-related health problems, and addictions. They are:

Stage 1—Precontemplation (denial):
Attitude: "I don't need to lose weight" or "I don't think I could ever lose weight."
Stage 2—Contemplation:
Attitude: "I think I need to lose weight. I wonder what I can do."
Stage 3—Planning:
Attitude: "I am going to lose weight and this is how I will do it."
Stage 4—Action:
Attitude: "I am on a weight-loss program and I am going to stick it out."
Stage 5—Maintenance and recovery from relapse:
Attitude: "I have lost weight and I am going to keep it off" or "I've had a slip and gained a bit of weight back, but I know what to do and I am going to get back on track."

What stage are you at in your readiness to change? If you are in pre-contemplation or denial (Stage 1), you are probably not yet ready for change. If you are overweight, perhaps your doctor needs to give you a wake-up call and help you to understand what health problems you will likely face if you don't get your weight under control. If you are hovering in the contemplation stage (Stage 2), you might be reading different diet books or dabbling with different weight-loss approaches. For serious results, you have to study this program thoroughly and get ready to put it into action. In the meantime, making small changes like learning to eat more volumetric foods, taking PGX, avoiding desserts and second helpings, and reducing portion sizes can help you pave the way to success.

In our experience, those who achieve the greatest success are those who study the principles of this program and carefully plan (Stage 3), put this program into action (Stage 4), and then maintain (Stage 5). Set a date for your program to begin officially and plan to make a commitment for real and lasting change. If you are indeed ready for change, the Hunger Free Forever program will help you achieve lifelong weight control comfortably and with minimal sacrifice.

Seven Keys to Successful Change

1. Make both short-term and long-term goals.
2. Know what you need to do and what you need to avoid to achieve change.
3. Ask for support from family and friends.
4. Have realistic expectations.
5. Stay motivated even if you don't see immediate results.
6. Recognize that change can be difficult, but you must stay the course.
7. Believe that you really can change.

WEIGHT-LOSS SUCCESS HABIT #1: TAILOR YOUR FOOD PORTIONS

Learning to reduce portion sizes for higher calorie foods while increasing portion sizes of low-caloric density, volumetric foods is critical for long-term success. Because portion sizes have increased substantially over the last few years, most people have little idea what an appropriate portion of most foods really should look like. However, there is an easy tool for you to use—your hands. They can be used for a convenient portion guide.

An appropriate portion of lean meat or other high-protein food in a main meal during weight loss would be about the size of your palm and the thickness of your finger. When a 24-ounce sirloin is what you

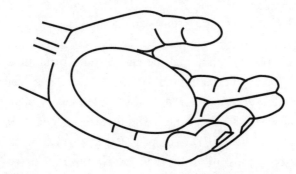

Figure 5.1. Meat, eggs, tofu or other lean protein foods = palm-size portion.

consider to be a normal portion of meat, reducing your portions to this smaller size will take some getting used to, but it is all your body really needs. For the healthiest protein portion possible, trim the visible fat from meats, remove the skin from poultry, and use cooking methods such as roasting, baking, or poaching that require little or no added fat. Avoid luncheon meats, sausages, and prepackaged meats. If you do eat these, choose those free of nitrates and lower in salt (sodium) and fat.

An appropriate portion of whole-grain bread or pasta, potatoes, yams, or other starchy vegetables would be about the size of your fist. Boiled whole grains, such as brown rice, wild rice, barley, or oatmeal are higher in volume and viscosity because they are rich in fiber and high in water, so it is always preferable to choose these starchy foods over less volumetric starchy foods such as white-flour pasta, white bread, and other white-flour products.

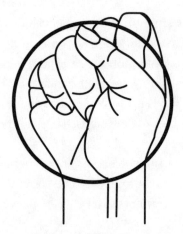

Figure 5.2. Starchy foods = fist-size portion.

High-fat foods, such as high-fat cheeses, chocolate, nuts, nut butters, and seeds should be limited to portions the size of your thumb. Pure fat foods, such as butter and other added fats or oils, including the oil in salad dressings or sauces, should be limited to about the size of the tip of your thumb. Do not avoid fats and oils altogether, but be sure to exercise moderation. Try to include healthy fats every day. Nuts and seeds, olive oil, and fish oils are examples of fats that you should eat regularly.

Pure fats and oils ⎯⎯⎯⟶

High fat foods ⎯⎯⎯⟶

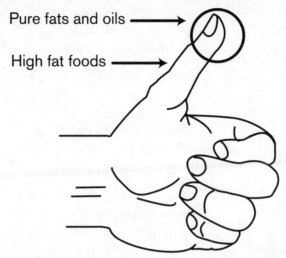

Figure 5.3. Pure fats and oils = tip of thumb portion. High-fat foods such as cheese, chocolate, nuts, and seeds = whole thumb portion.

Nonstarchy vegetables, including salads and cooked vegetables (steamed, grilled, baked, stir-fried, or added to various cooked dishes) should be eaten in abundance. An appropriate portion would be the amount you can hold in both hands; however, more can be eaten if desired or needed to control appetite. Avoid cream sauces and use oily salad dressings sparingly with these vegetables. Many low-fat recipes for making delicious vegetables are provided in chapter 10.

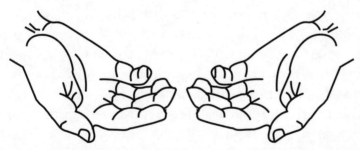

Figure 5.4. Cooked and raw nonstarchy vegetables = two hand-fuls (or more) portion size.

Finally, a portion of fruit or a portion of a low-fat milk or dairy product (like plain yogurt) should be about the size of one fist. These

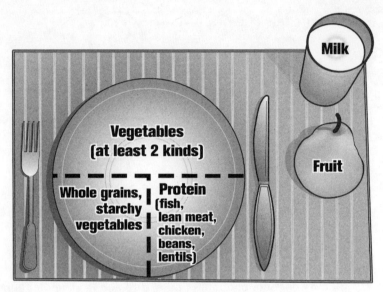

Figure 5.5. A Portion-Controlled Plate.

foods can be included in a balanced meal or can be used as hunger-reducing snacks or desserts.

Are You a Victim of Portion Distortion?

Over the past few decades, most of us have become accustomed to eating more food than ever before. The average number of calories consumed by Americans has gone up thanks to a combination of increased portion sizes and an increased intake of high caloric–density foods. According to USDA data, the average American was eating 523 calories more per day in 2003 than in 1970, or enough calories to add about 50 pounds of fat per year to each American. Obviously, not many people are gaining 50 pounds per year, but a tendency to eat more calories than we need is a problem facing nearly everyone in America as well as every other developed country.

Bit by bit, portion sizes have increased in restaurants, packaged foods, and on our dinner plates. Food companies have long known that people want to get value for their money and simply giving consumers more food is the easiest way to keep people coming back to a restaurant or a food product. Fat, sugar, and refined flour also sell food,

U.S. AVERAGE DAILY CALORIC INTAKE: 1970–2003

From 1970 to 2003 the average daily caloric intake grew by 523 calories
Per capita consumption of Americans (USDA Data*)

Commodity group	1970	2003	Increase in pounds, 1970–2003	Increase in daily calories, 1970–2003
	Pounds		*Percent*	*Number*
Fats and oils	53	86	63	216
Grains	136	194	43	188
Sugar and sweeteners	119	142	19	76
Meat, eggs, and nuts	226	242	7	24
Vegetables	337	418	24	16
Fruits	242	275	12	14
Dairy	564	594	5	-11
Total	1,675	1,950	16% (almost 300 lbs/yr)	523 calories/day

* The USDA per capita data represent the amount of food and calories available for consumption after adjusting for spoilage, plate waste, and other losses in the home or marketing system.

so these ingredients have gone up disproportionately to portion sizes, thus increasing the average caloric density of foods. Learning to eat more volumetric foods while limiting portions of higher caloric–density foods is the best strategy to overcome this portion distortion.

Are Your Eyes Bigger Than Your Stomach?

We have all used the saying "my eyes were bigger than my stomach" when we piled more food on our plate than we could eat. However, research has actually shown that your eyes determine the size of your stomach. Several studies have demonstrated that people will eat more food when more food is put in front of them, and yet feel no more satisfied than if they ate less. In other words, if you pile large portions of food on a big plate, you won't tend to feel full until you have eaten much more food than if you were to put smaller portions of food on a smaller plate. Your eyes play a significant role in telling your brain how much food you need to feel full.

The reality is that modern-day portion sizes are so large that you could easily cut most portions in half or even one-third and still eat enough food to feel easily satisfied. The key to getting used to smaller portion sizes is to be sure that you consume larger portions of volumetric foods that are high in fiber and water first, then eat smaller portions of the higher calorie elements of your meal more slowly.

Practicing Portion Control

Portion control can take some time to master, but it is a skill that is completely necessary for long-term weight control. If you balance your food selections correctly, you will never have to feel hungry, even when you are losing weight. If you significantly increase your vegetable and fruit intake, and reduce your fat intake to a very modest level, portion control over other foods will be relatively simple. In addition, consuming PGX before, during, or after meals is another strategy to bring about satiety while decreasing portion sizes. Five grams of PGX will hold about one liter of water as it passes through the stomach and small intestine. Since most people's stomachs holds about two liters of water, a 5-gram serving of PGX prior to your meal will allow you to cut your portion sizes easily in half and still have the sensation of feeling full.

Eating out is a particular challenge for those who want to lose weight, but even eating out can add to your success if you practice careful portion control. One important key is to order a dinner-size salad to start, with the dressing on the side. Discard all of the croutons and other high-calorie bits, then dip your fork in the dressing before you pick up the salad. This adds enough flavor to make the salad enjoyable and you will only use a small amount of dressing by the time you finish the salad. Then, since the main course usually contains two to three times more food than you need, eat only half your meal and take the other half home for lunch the next day. One good habit is to ask the server to put half of your main course in a takeout box even before it comes to the table. As an alternative, you can split a main course with a friend, or have a low-fat, low-calorie main course such as broiled fish and only eat a small portion of the rice or potatoes. You can also ask for substitutions. For example, ask for steamed vegetables instead of french fries, extra salad instead of rice. Be sure to ask for all sauces, butter, dressings, and gravy on the side and use them sparingly.

WEIGHT-LOSS SUCCESS HABIT #2: TAKE YOUR TIME WHEN EATING

Before you eat, your digestive system speaks to your brain through nerve and chemical signals to increase your feelings of hunger. When you eat, your digestive system continues to carry on a dialogue with your brain, eventually leading to a sense of fullness and a termination of your meal. But unfortunately, it can take a full twenty minutes for your brain to get the message that you've eaten enough food.

Research has shown that most people with weight problems eat quicker and swallow significantly more food in the same period of time as people with normal weight. The overweight person has a tendency to eat bite after bite of food in rapid succession, easily overeating before they even begin to feel that they have had enough. Certainly, one of the simplest and most effective strategies for losing weight is to practice eating slowly and learning to savor every bite. If you can truly master the art of eating slowly and mindfully, you can dramatically decrease the size of the portions you eat and still feel wonderfully satisfied with every meal.

Although this may seem like common sense, and a fairly simple thing to do, many overweight people have such compulsive eating patterns that they will continually forget this principle and halfway through their meal realize that they have been wolfing down their food once again. However, there is good news. In our clinical experience, we have found some simple but very effective keys to slow down the overweight eater:.

- Never sit down to eat a main meal when you are too hungry. Learn to "spoil your appetite" with healthy snacks before each meal. Or take 2.5 to 5 grams of PGX before meals (three to six PGX softgel capsules, one to two SlimStyles capsules, a half to one scoop of PGX granules).

- Start the meal with a large volumetric salad or soup. These starters take some time to eat and that takes the edge off your appetite, giving your stomach a chance to let the brain know that you have eaten nearly enough food.

- Put your fork or spoon down after every bite. For many people, eating is a nonstop motion: The fork or spoon is racing from plate to mouth. Instead, take a small spoonful of food, then put the spoon down beside your plate while you chew your food thoroughly. Don't pick up the spoon until you have completely swallowed the previous bite.

- Pause after eating the first half of your meal and allow yourself a few minutes to feel satiated. You just may find you're too full to eat the other half anyway. Carry on a conversation and give your stomach time to register the food you have eaten.

- Sit down to eat your meals and snacks, but don't sit down in front of the television. If you eat your main meals or snacks while watching TV, you are likely to lose your focus, leading to mindless munching.

- Don't eat seconds or thirds. If you are still hungry or tempted to eat after your meal, eat some raw vegetables or an apple, or drink a large glass of water with PXG fiber.

IS THERE A PLACE FOR SMOOTHIES AND MEAL REPLACEMENTS IN LONG-TERM WEIGHT CONTROL?

Eating slowly and mindfully is one of the most important ways to promote satiety and avoid eating too much food. However, high-protein volumetric smoothies and high-protein meal replacement beverages are still invaluable in short-term weight loss as well as long-term weight maintenance. Many people simply don't have time to prepare three meals per day and end up skipping meals or eating unhealthy snack foods instead. Meal replacement beverages and smoothies can provide a high-satiety, quick meal that will stay with you for hours and give you a highly nutritious alternative to fast food or unhealthy snack foods.

Numerous studies have shown that meal replacements can play

an important role not only in weight loss, but in long-term weight maintenance. At our center, we make extensive use of meal replacement beverages containing full servings of PGX and high-quality whey protein (see www.PGX.com and www.Slimstyles.com for examples of meal replacements containing PGX). These ingredients promote satiety and make these products superior to typical meal replacements like SlimFast. (Hint: Adding 2.5 to 5 grams of PGX granules to a serving of SlimFast will transform it into a high-satiety snack.) We also make sure our patients are skilled at making high-protein blender smoothies with added PGX and whey protein. Replacing one or two meals per day with a high-protein blender smoothie or meal replacement beverage can leave you with the time and energy to focus on your other meals and can help you to lose weight simply and comfortably.

WEIGHT-LOSS SUCCESS HABIT #3: THINK AHEAD AND PLAN WHAT YOU ARE GOING TO EAT

Humans plan; animals act on impulse. One of the principal reasons why weight problems have become so prevalent is that our fast-paced way of life leads us to act on our animal instincts when it comes to food. Unfortunately, eating on the run and grabbing food on impulse promotes wrong food choices that can easily pack on extra calories. If you eat when your appetite is in overdrive and you stop at the drive-through or raid the refrigerator, you tend to choose the tastiest food rather than what is most sensible.

Eating on impulse makes you more like an animal with little regard to the consequences of your actions, and less like a human with wisdom and intelligence behind your decisions. Think what would happen if you gave your dog a choice between a cheeseburger, fries, and a milkshake or dry dog food and water. Of course, most dogs would impulsively choose the tasty fast food and would completely ignore their nutritious dog food. If they were allowed to make this impulsive choice day after day, they would invariably become obese and die prematurely. Of course, we are all smarter than dogs, but if you want to get your weight under control, you must develop some nutritional wisdom and avoid impulse eating at all costs. Fortunately, with some easily acquired knowledge and a bit of planning, impulse eating can be a thing of the past.

Twenty Minutes for a Healthier You

Even the busiest people can find the time to do a bit of planning and add some structure to their eating habits. We encourage our patients to sit down before the week begins, usually on Sunday night, and plan out what they're going to eat for the week. A simple menu plan with seven breakfasts, lunches, and dinners along with healthy snacks, can be easily accomplished in about twenty minutes. From this menu plan, a grocery list can be easily compiled.

Well-planned meals don't need to take a lot of time. There are thousands of recipes that require only minutes of preparation and little culinary skill. Salads are, of course, a staple in any weight-loss program. It is well worth your while to learn a few good ways to make tasty, high-volume, low-calorie salads in a flash. Also, making huge pots of high-volume, low-calorie soup and freezing small portions that can be thawed in minutes is another way to have instant high-satiety meals on hand.

If you plan properly, your fridge and pantry will always have plenty of healthy foods that can be eaten in an instant or prepared in seconds. Always be sure that you have plenty of healthy snacks like pears, berries, carrots, cucumbers, plain yogurt, hard-boiled eggs, nonfat cheese, and oatmeal that will give you plenty of options when you don't have time to prepare something and you want to avoid eating high-calorie foods on impulse. Always having ingredients for healthy smoothies such as frozen fruit and whey protein, or having weight-loss meal replacement drinks on hand can also fill the gap when you need good nutrition and just can't afford the time to prepare a meal.

Menu Planning with Your Computer

The Internet can make meal planning very easy. There are numerous Web sites that have hundreds or even thousands of recipes, many of which can be used very successfully as part of a weight-loss program. Some of these sites enable you to create your own personal cookbooks with the recipes you want to try; they often have features that allow you to create a menu plan and shopping list in seconds. The site that we recommend is www.RecipeZaar.com. It has about 200,000 user-contributed recipes, many of which are rated by users and have accompanying pictures. Using this resource, you can quickly compile your personal weight-loss cookbook. Within a few minutes, you can plan out your whole week's meals and generate a shopping list.

Today, many people have little knowledge or limited skills when it comes to preparing even simple foods from scratch. Fortunately, with resources like the Internet and numerous cooking channels, you can become quite competent in healthy food preparation in very little time if you are willing to commit to learning a few new techniques.

Planning for Eating Out

For most people, eating out is an unavoidable way of life. Business travel, frequent meetings, and just sheer lack of time and energy make it very difficult to avoid eating out on a regular basis. However, if you want to lose weight and keep it off over the long haul, try to eat out less. When you do decide to eat out, be sure to determine in advance that you are going to make wise food choices and keep on track with your weight-loss program. Choosing a restaurant wisely and knowing what is on the restaurant's menu can help you decide what you are going to eat before you arrive and are tempted and begin to be influenced by all of the wonderful aromas. In addition, remember to always try to spoil your appetite by eating something healthy or taking PGX before you get to the restaurant to avoid being overly tempted to choose the higher calorie menu items. Most restaurants, even fast-food joints, offer a variety of healthy salads and other low-calorie items so it is easily possible to eat out, make wise food choices, and still enjoy yourself.

WEIGHT-LOSS SUCCESS HABIT #4: TURN TO DELICIOUS HEALTHY FOODS AND TURN AWAY FROM PROBLEM FOODS

Dieting for weight loss usually means depriving yourself of delicious food. Because food is so central to our enjoyment of life, few people can stick to a diet. At our clinical research center, rather than getting people to diet, we encourage people to discover a wide range of foods that are delicious and yet are completely in keeping with their weight-loss goals.

Several years ago, researchers at the National Institutes of Health wanted to understand why it was so difficult to get people with high cholesterol or heart disease to lower their cholesterol through dietary change. What they discovered was that people could not endure a diet when the emphasis was placed on foods that they had to avoid. So the researchers switched gears and focused on teaching people to prepare and eat foods that were delicious but still in line with a diet that would lower cholesterol. They found that when people were able to eat foods that they completely enjoyed, they had no difficulty remaining faithful to the diet. By focusing on what they could enjoy, rather than on what they had to avoid, they achieved dieting success.

Turn to Delicious Healthy Foods

We have used this principle for many years in helping our patients to lose weight and reverse diabetes and cardiac risk factors. We have seen in hundreds of cases that if people can discover a repertoire of meals and snacks that they completely enjoy, they can easily steer away from foods and snacks that will sabotage their weight-loss goals.

Some of the simpler foods in this program are not favorites at first, but become favorites as your taste buds adapt to more simple flavors. For example, apples are a simple food that most of our weight-loss patients eat every day. If you have a sweet tooth, apples may not taste that great at first, but if you persist in eating apples, it isn't too long before an apple becomes a delicious sweet treat. Likewise, raw vegetables may even turn your stomach at first if you eat them by themselves. You'll probably need to find a few healthy dips and dressings to make eating raw vegetables enjoyable. However, as time goes on, you'll enjoy raw vegetables more and more. There are also hundreds of ways to thoroughly enjoy vegetables roasted, grilled, steamed, stir-fried, and cooked into soups and stews.

If you want to improve your diet radically and make your weight-loss efforts easy and enjoyable, invest the time and effort in discovering foods and recipes that you can enjoy and still stick with your weight-loss goals. With just a few good recipes and snacks, such as those provided in chapter 10, you are well on your way to changing your diet without feeling deprivation.

Turn Away from Problem Foods

Although this program emphasizes good-tasting foods that assist in your weight-loss goals, it is important to realize that there are foods that can easily sabotage your success if you don't learn to turn away from them. Does this mean that you can never eat chocolate or ice cream? No. As long as you are able to eat these foods in real moderation and on an infrequent basis, they pose no real problem. For example, many people can eat a very small square of chocolate one tiny nibble at a time and not end up eating many extra calories. Others, however, would be better off abstaining from chocolate altogether because they are unable to be moderate in their consumption. If they eat one tiny piece, it inflames their passions and they end up eating several hundred calories of chocolate before they are able to stop.

When it comes to problem foods, our guidelines are the same as those we give for alcohol consumption. For example, moderate drinkers can have one or two drinks and they are perfectly happy to stop. There is no inner compulsion that drives them to drink more and more after that first drink. An alcoholic, on the other hand, is far better off abstaining from alcohol altogether. For an alcoholic, one or two drinks tend to turn on compulsive desires that lead them to drink to excess. In the same way, many overweight people find greater success in maintaining abstinence from high-calorie, super tasty foods rather than trying to exert self-control over these high temptation choices.

Should you abstain from certain foods, or are you able to maintain careful moderation? This question is one you need to answer honestly for

A FEW FOODS THAT CAN MAKE YOU FAT REAL FAST
- Ice cream
- Cookies, cakes, pies
- Donuts and pastries
- White bread and white-flour products
- Cheese (except low-fat versions)
- Mayonnaise (except low-fat versions)
- Fried foods, especially deep fried
- White sugar, chocolate, candy
- Pop, fruit juice, and other sugary drinks
- Bacon, sausage, wieners, processed meats
- Hot dogs, fast-food burgers
- Potato chips and tortilla chips
- White rice
- Sugary breakfast cereals

yourself. Fortunately, if you follow the principles of the Hunger Free Forever program, unhealthy food cravings vanish or are greatly diminished, making it easier to turn away from problem foods. Alternately, if you suspect you have a food addiction, see "Food as a Drug" on facing page.

WEIGHT-LOSS SUCCESS HABIT #5: TAKE TIME TO CULTIVATE HEALTHY HABITS AND TERMINATE BAD HABITS AND FOOD ADDICTIONS

Are you tripped up by destructive habits? If you have a weight problem, you undoubtedly have certain habits that work against your desire to achieve and maintain an ideal body weight. Perhaps bad eating habits are the primary reason why you fail in your weight-loss efforts or why you gain weight back after successfully losing weight. Eating to relieve stress, boredom, or depression; compulsively overeating as a brief escape from reality; or eating impulsively because you just don't care about the consequences, are just of few of the self-destructive habits that so commonly sabotage a person's desire to lose weight.

What is it that allows for such lapses in good judgment and self-restraint when, in our heart, we really want to respect our bodies and get our weight under control? In reality, habit is a powerful force, good or bad, and a force that needs to be directed for our benefit rather than for our destruction. If we ignore our bad habits or just try to cover them over with willpower, they will always come back to haunt us.

The Nature of Habit and Addiction

Habits are formed when we repeat certain behaviors so often that they eventually become a learned behavior or a program within the brain. In fact, habits actually reflect changes in the structure of the brain that is modified with thousands of new nerve cell branches and connections as the habit becomes stronger. In essence, learned behaviors, whether they are a new skill or an addiction, become an easily repeated pattern of brain activity that is literally hard-wired into the brain. The appetite centers located in the hypothalamus of the brain are particularly "plastic," meaning that nerve pathways into and out of this region can be significantly rewired by repetitive eating behaviors. In this way, bad eating habits can eventually become a natural and normal experience that is very hard to stop by willpower alone.

Fortunately, the neural plasticity of the brain's appetite centers means that practicing better eating behaviors can also result in rewiring the brain so that these healthier behaviors can become as natural and pleasant as the unhealthy behaviors you are replacing. When you are freed from an appetite in overdrive with the Hunger Free Forever program, you can begin to practice better eating habits with minimal sacrifice and no discomfort. If you persist in repeating these healthy behaviors, in a few weeks these better habits will become second nature.

Food as a Drug

Unfortunately, many people with weight problems use food as a drug, and many have food behaviors that can be properly classified as addictive behaviors—compulsive, self-destructive habits for which the addict has little control. You can't underestimate the potential potency of food as an addictive substance. Food stimulates powerful feelings of pleasure, feelings that are normal and healthy. However, if people begin to use wrong food choices or excesses of food to mask their pain and to escape from reality, they may end up struggling with their eating habits much like someone addicted to cocaine.

Addictions or self-destructive habits are learned behaviors that result in the experience of pleasures and relief of discomfort. Once an addiction is formed, it becomes a permanent part of the brain's structure. This is why, for instance, alcoholism is a treatable but not curable disease. Alcoholics who no longer drink properly refer to themselves as alcoholics in recovery, rather than ex-alcoholics, even if they have been sober for decades. If the alcoholic begins to drink again, the old brain circuits come back to life very quickly, and they usually become compulsive drinkers soon after that. Likewise, people who have overcome obesity are really "recovering" obese people who have the potential to fall back into their old patterns again unless they carefully manage their eating behaviors.

How to Overcome Self-Defeating Eating Habits

At our center, we teach a simple approach to habit change that has been used successfully since the 1970s by experts in behavior modification around the world. This approach, known as habit reversal ther-

ARE YOU ADDICTED TO FOOD?

Bad eating habits and minor food addictions are common and relatively easy to change in most people with weight problems using the simple behavior modification methods we discuss in this chapter. However, a small minority of the overweight or obese, particularly those with severe weight problems, need special support and counseling of a nature similar to the support given to alcoholics and other chemically dependent people. At our center, in addition to following the Hunger Free Forever program, we recommend that these people get involved with Overeaters Anonymous, an international nonprofit support group network that follows the same 12-step program used and respected in addiction treatment centers around the world. Overeaters Anonymous has branches across North America and in many other parts of the world. For more information, see www.OA.org.

apy, was developed and has been used extensively to help individuals troubled with serious compulsive behaviors such as stuttering, as well as various addictions such as to nicotine. We have adapted this method to those with weight problems and find it to be highly successful in helping people to overcome self-defeating eating habits. This approach involves three important steps:

1. Increase awareness of the bad habit.
2. Find a harmless or healthy habit to replace the bad habit.
3. Reduce stress levels and feelings of depression.

Increase Awareness of the Bad Habit

Increasing awareness of the bad habit starts by keeping a detailed food record for several days. During this time, you eat the kinds and quantities of food that you usually do, including all bad eating habits—for example, snacking on high-calorie foods after dinner or eating more than one helping of food for dinner. It is important to record the time and quantity of every food you eat, including all snacks, and everything you drink.

At our center, we have patients review their food records with a registered dietician. If you can get the help of a dietician this is ideal, but if not, you will find it helpful to spend time carefully keeping and then reviewing your own food record. Most people are unaware of or forget about 30 percent of the calories they eat. Keeping food records for several days and repeating this on a regular basis helps to increase your awareness of your food habits and the foods that you eat mindlessly. You can't overcome your bad habits if you aren't crystal clear about the full nature of these habits. Weighing yourself and measuring your waist circumference frequently is another way to monitor your eating behavior and to catch yourself early on if your weight starts to go up. Rather than hovering in denial, you can get back to action and keep your weight-loss goals.

Find a Harmless or Healthy Habit to Replace the Bad Habit

Rather than just trying to stop cold when you feel like repeating the bad habit, substitute a harmless or healthy behavior. For instance, if you have the bad habit of eating a sweet, high-calorie dessert after supper, eat an apple or a few carrots when you get this urge. Your brain will adapt to this new behavior and accept it as a suitable replacement for the bad habit more easily than if you tried to eat nothing. Likewise, if you find yourself snacking all evening, you are better off nibbling on fresh fruit, raw vegetables, or a pudding made with a PGX-containing meal replacement instead of just trying to stop eating during the evening. Substituting a good habit for a bad habit is easier and will be more successful than just trying to stop the old bad behavior. The brain program that controls your bad habit will adapt and accept the new healthier habit as an acceptable response to the unhealthy impulse to eat. In essence, the old program will never go away, but it can be shaped and programmed into something good for you. This is why habit substitution is much more successful than just trying to stop a bad habit.

Reduce Stress Levels and Feelings of Depression

Finally, reducing stress levels and feelings of depression can play an important role in terminating bad eating habits. Stress, depression, loneliness, and boredom can all be powerful triggers to stimulate inappropriate eating. If you are using food as a drug or an escape from stress, you need to find healthier ways to reduce your stress. A commitment to regular exercise and learning stress management techniques can really increase the success of your weight-loss efforts. If your unhealthy eating habits are triggered by feelings of depression, emptiness, or loneliness, you may need to seek professional or spiritual help to get at the root of your problems. Food cannot cure a wounded or empty soul.

Letting Habits Work for You

We have learned over the years that success breeds success. If you begin with the simplest parts of this program, your appetite will be reduced, your blood sugar stabilized, and you will likely be able to make significant progress in your quest toward an ideal body weight. Setting realistic goals that can be achieved within reasonable amounts of time is a good place to start. We normally recommend people set their initial weight loss goal to be 5 to 10 percent of their current weight. Once you have achieved this goal, your initial success will stimulate confidence as you realize that this first step was not all that difficult. Even if you lose weight slowly, if you continue to make changes that you can stick with, in the long run you can still achieve your weight-loss goals. After all, it would be far better to average a weight loss of 1 pound per month for four years and keep it off, than to lose 50 pounds in eight weeks and then gain it all back. It is important to condition yourself to accept changes in your eating habits and lifestyle that you can live with for the rest of your life.

CHAPTER SUMMARY

- The kind of food we eat, when we eat, how fast, and how much we eat are all choices and behaviors that need to be aligned with our weight-loss goals if we want to achieve long-term success.
- The five key habits critical to support a lifetime of healthy weight are:
  1. Tailor your food portions.
  2. Take your time when eating.
  3. Think ahead and plan what you are going to eat.
  4. Turn to delicious, healthy foods and turn away from problem foods.
  5. Take time to cultivate healthy habits and terminate bad habits and food addictions.
- Habit reversal therapy can be a very effective therapy for defeating eating problems.
- It is important to condition yourself to accept changes in your eating habits and lifestyle that you can live with for the rest of your life.

6

REDUCE THE EFFECTS OF
STRESS AND CORTISOL

Everyday stress is a normal part of modern living. Job pressures, family arguments, financial pressures, traffic, and time management are just a few of the stressors we are faced with on a daily basis. However, technically speaking, a stressor may be almost any disturbance—heat or cold, a stormy day, environmental toxins, toxins produced by microorganisms, physical trauma, and strong emotional reactions—that can trigger a number of biological changes to produce what is commonly known as the stress response.

Fortunately for us, control mechanisms in the body are geared toward counteracting the everyday stresses of life. Most often the stress response is so mild that it goes entirely unnoticed. However, if stress is extreme, unusual, or long-lasting, the stress response can be overwhelming and quite harmful.

One of the consequences of the stress response is abdominal fat cell growth and loss of muscle mass, a scenario that leads to insulin resistance and obesity. The adrenal hormone cortisol, released as a result of the stress response, is ultimately responsible for the fact that stress promotes weight gain because it promotes insulin resistance and raises blood sugar levels.

In this chapter, we detail a comprehensive stress management program designed to counteract the everyday stresses of life and reset proper appetite control and metabolism by reducing excessive cortisol secretion. But before we can discuss methods for helping you deal more effectively with stress and lower cortisol levels, we need to explain the underlying features of the stress response and how it contributes to obesity.

STRESS: A HEALTHY VIEW

So often we think of stress as a negative in our lives, but stress is actually a good thing. Dr. Hans Selye, the Canadian researcher and father of modern stress research, developed valuable insights into the role of stress in our lives. According to Selye, stress in itself should not be viewed in a negative context. It is not the stressor that determines the response; instead it is the individual's internal reaction, which then triggers the response. This internal reaction is highly individualized and holds the real key to the effects of stress. What one person may experience as stress, the next person may view as exhilirating. Selye perhaps summarized his view best in the following passage from his book, *The Stress of Life*:

> No one can live without experiencing some degree of stress all the time. You may think that only serious disease or intensive physical or mental injury can cause stress. This is false. Crossing a busy intersection, exposure to a draft, or even sheer joy are enough to activate the body's stress mechanisms to some extent. Stress is not even necessarily bad for you; it is also the spice of life, for any emotion, any activity causes stress, but, of course, your system must be prepared to take it. The same stress which makes one person sick can be an invigorating experience for another.

The key statement Selye made is "your system must be prepared to take [stress]." That is the crux of this chapter—to help you understand how you can strengthen your resistance to stress by giving your body and mind the support that it needs.

THE STRESS RESPONSE

If you have ever been suddenly frightened, you definitely know what the stress response feels like when it is fully engaged. The initial response to stress is called the fight-or-flight response. It is actually just the first phase of a larger response known as the general adaptation syndrome. The three phases of the general adaptation syndrome are: alarm, resistance, and exhaustion. These phases are largely controlled and regulated by the adrenal glands, a small organ that sits on top of each kidney, which are the source of adrenaline, cortisol, and other key hormones involved in the stress response.

Although the alarm phase is usually a short-lived rush of adrenaline, the next phase—the *resistance reaction*—allows the body to continue fighting a stressor long after the effects of the fight-or-flight response have worn off. The adrenal hormone cortisol is largely responsible for the resistance reaction. The effects of cortisol are quite necessary when the body is faced with danger, but prolongation of the resistance reaction or continued stress sets the stage for weight gain and increases the risk of significant diseases including diabetes, high blood pressure, and cancer.

Extreme or prolonged stress results in the final stage of the general adaptation syndrome, exhaustion, which may manifest as a partial or total collapse of a body function or specific organ. Two of the major causes of exhaustion are loss of potassium ions and depletion of adrenal hormones like DHEA and cortisol. Loss of potassium results in cellular dysfunction and, if it is severe, cell death. Lower levels of DHEA and cortisol are associated with extreme fatigue, impaired blood sugar control, and a diminished response to stress. While the entire body is affected by prolonged stress, the heart, blood vessels, adrenals, and immune system are affected the most. Not surprising, prolonged stress and poor stress management are associated with many common diseases.

CONDITIONS LINKED TO STRESS

Angina	High blood pressure
Asthma	Irritable bowel syndrome (IBS)
Autoimmune disease	Lowered immunity
Cancer	Menstrual irregularities
Cardiovascular disease	Nonulcer dyspepsia
Colds	Obesity
Depression	Rheumatoid arthritis
Diabetes (type 2)	Ulcerative colitis
Headaches	Ulcers

SIDE EFFECTS OF EXCESSIVE CORTISOL

Elevated cortisol levels are associated with increased appetite, cravings for sugar, and weight gain. To appreciate the full effect of excessive cortisol secretion on our physiology, let's take a look at the well-known side effects of a drug form of cortisol, prednisone. Used primarily in allergic and inflammatory conditions like asthma and rheumatoid arthritis, prednisone is by far the most often prescribed oral corticosteroid. It blocks many key steps in the allergic and inflammatory response, including the production and secretion of compounds that promote inflammation by white blood cells. This disruption of the normal defense functions of the white blood cells is great at stopping the inflammatory response, but it essentially cripples the immune system. Long-term use of prednisone also causes abdominal obesity, puffiness of the face ("moon face"), and accumulation of fat in the upper back ("buffalo hump").

The side effects of prednisone relate to dosage levels and length of time on the drug. Most of the side effects are not due to taking too much of the drug for a short period of time, but rather are due to long-term use, even at lower dosages. At lower doses (less than 10 mg per day) the most notable side effects are usually increased appetite, weight gain, retention of salt and water, and increased susceptibility to infection.

Common side effects of long-term prednisone use at higher dosage levels include: depression, insomia, mood swings, personality changes and even psychotic behavior; high blood pressure; diabetes; peptic ulcers; acne; excessive facial hair in women; muscle cramps and weakness; thinning and weakening of the skin; osteoporosis; and susceptibility to the formation of blood clots. Unfortunately, every single one of prednisone's side effects, both short- and long-term, can occur in our bodies due to excessive cortisol secretion.

Cortisol, Visceral Fat, and Appetite

Cortisol exerts a double whammy on fat cells in the abdomen: 1) it stimulates their growth; and 2) it stimulates the manufacture of new abdominal fat cells. So not only does cortisol signal the brain to eat more, it increases the amount of visceral (abdominal) fat. As you will recall, when visceral fat increases, it leads to the release of hormones that block the action of insulin and promote the appetite.

Cortisol also adversely affects appetite and promotes the craving of carbohydrates by lowering brain serotonin levels. Serotonin is an important brain chemical that promotes a sense of relaxation and positive mood (happiness). When your brain is low in serotonin, carbohydrate cravings result. What the brain is trying to accomplish by signaling a carbohydrate craving is increasing the manufacture of serotonin from the amino acid tryptophan. Tryptophan has a difficult time getting into the brain because it competes with other amino acids for transport across the blood-brain barrier. After a high-carbohydrate meal, there are fewer molecules of amino acids that compete with tryptophan circulating in the bloodstream, thanks to our friend insulin. While insulin's primary job is to remove sugar from the blood and help it pass into the cells, it also promotes the absorption of certain amino acids into muscle tissue. As a result, there are fewer amino acids to compete with tryptophan for transport through the blood-brain barrier. Therefore, as long as cortisol levels are high, leading to low brain serotonin levels, carbohydrate cravings will be strong.

5-HYDROXYTRYPTOPHAN (5-HTP), SATIETY, AND WEIGHT LOSS

The amino acid 5-HTP is the intermediate step between tryptophan and the important brain chemical serotonin. Trytophan is converted to 5-HTP, which in turn is converted into serotonin. Cortisol lowers brain serotonin levels because it inhibits the conversion of tryptophan to 5-HTP. As a result, many people with high stress levels are overweight, crave sugar and other carbohydrates, experience bouts of depression, get frequent headaches, and have vague muscle aches and pains. All of these maladies are correctable by raising brain serotonin levels with 5-HTP.

5-HTP VERSUS TRYPTOPHAN: A COMPARISON

Research has shown that, by all measures, supplemental 5-HTP is far superior to supplemental L-tryptophan for boosting serotonin levels. Here are some of the reasons why:

- Commercially available 5-HTP that has been extracted from a natural source, the seed of an African plant known as *Griffonia simplicifolia*, is not vulnerable to contamination. One process by which L-tryptophan is manufactured involves fermentation of bacteria, which does pose a risk of contamination.
- 5-HTP, unlike L-tryptophan, cannot be metabolized by the liver into kynurenine—a substance that in turn inhibits the conversion of tryptophan to 5-HTP, hence producing lower serotonin levels.
- While about 70 percent of a dose of 5-HTP taken orally is delivered to the bloodstream for transport to the brain for conversion to serotonin, only about 3 percent of a dose of L-trytophan is eventually converted into serotonin.
- 5-HTP passes into the brain immediately, while tryptophan must compete with other proteins to be transported across the blood-brain barrier.
- 5-HTP raises levels of other brain neurotransmitters, including melatonin, dopamine, and norepinephrine. L-tryptophan does not have this effect.

5-HTP as a Weight-Loss Aid

As far back as 1975, researchers demonstrated that administering 5-HTP to rats that were bred to overeat and be obese resulted in significant reduction in food intake. It turns out that these rats had decreased activity of the enzyme that converts tryptophan to 5-HTP and subsequently to serotonin. In other words, these rats were fat as a result of a genetically determined low level of activity of the enzyme that starts the manufacture of serotonin from tryptophan. As a result, the rats never got the message to stop eating until they had consumed far greater amounts of food than normal rats.

There is much circumstantial evidence that many humans are genetically predisposed to obesity. This predisposition may involve the same mechanism as that observed in the rats. In other words, many people may be predisposed to being overweight because they have a decreased conversion of tryptophan to 5-HTP and, as a result, decreased serotonin levels. By providing preformed 5-HTP, this genetic defect is bypassed and more serotonin is manufactured. In this way, 5-HTP literally turns off hunger.

The early animal studies that used 5-HTP as a weight-loss aid have been followed by a series of four human clinical studies of overweight women, conducted at the University of Rome. The first study showed that 5-HTP was able to reduce caloric intake and promote weight loss despite the fact that the women made no conscious effort to lose weight. The average amount of weight loss during the five-week period of 5-HTP supplementation was a little more than 3 pounds.

The second study sought to determine whether 5-HTP helped overweight individuals to adhere to dietary recommendations. The twelve-week study was divided into two six-week periods. For the first six weeks, there were no dietary recommendations; for the second six weeks, the women were placed on a 1,200-calorie diet. The women who took the placebo lost an average of 2.28 pounds, while the women who took the 5-HTP lost 10.34 pounds.

As in the previous study, 5-HTP appeared to promote weight loss by promoting satiety—the feeling of satisfaction—leading to fewer calories being consumed at meals. Every woman who took the 5-HTP reported early satiety.

In the third study involving 5-HTP, for the first six weeks there were no dietary restrictions, and for the second six weeks the women were placed on a 1,200-calorie-per-day diet. The results from this study were even more impressive than the previous studies for several reasons. The group that received the 5-HTP had lost an average of 4.39 pounds at six weeks and an average of 11.63 pounds at twelve weeks. In comparison, the placebo group had lost an average of only 0.62 pounds at six weeks and 1.87 pounds at twelve weeks. The lack of weight loss during the second six-week period in the placebo group obviously reflects the fact that the women had difficulty adhering to the diet.

Early satiety was reported by 100 percent of the subjects during the first six-week period. During the second six-week period, even with severe caloric restriction, 90 percent of the women taking 5-HTP reported early satiety. Many of the women who received the 5-HTP (300mg, three times per day) reported mild nausea during the first six weeks of therapy. However, the symptom was never severe enough for any of the women to drop out of the study. No other side effects were reported.

In the latest study, twenty-five overweight non-insulin dependent diabetic outpatients were enrolled in a double-blind, placebo-controlled study, and randomized to receive either 5-HTP (750mg per day) or a placebo for two consecutive weeks, during which no dietary restriction was prescribed. Results again indicated that patients receiving 5-HTP significantly decreased their daily energy intake by reducing carbohydrate and fat intake, and reduced their body weight.

While these studies used relatively high dosages of 5-HTP, our experience is that lower dosages of 50 to 100mg, twenty minutes before meals, are just as effective. We recommend 5-HTP only for those people who have intense carbohydrate cravings or who have other signs of low serotonin levels such as depressed mood. When taking a 5-HTP product, make sure that it is enteric coated, a process that prevents the breakdown of the capsule until it passes through the stomach. Nonenteric coated 5-HTP products can produce a great deal of stomach discomfort and nausea.

MANAGING STRESS

Whether you are aware of it or not, you definitely have developed a pattern for coping with stress. Unfortunately, most people have found patterns and methods that ultimately do not support good health. These include negative coping patterns such as overeating, uncontrolled emotional outbursts, feelings of helplessness, having a cocktail or beer, or smoking a cigarette. It is important for you to identify any negative coping pattern and replace it with positive ways of coping.

We believe that effective stress management involves three equally important areas:

• Techniques to calm the mind and promote a positive mental attitude
• Following a healthy lifestyle, including regular physical exercise
• Supporting your body by eating a healthful diet and utilizing key dietary and botanical supplements.

Calming the Mind and Body

Learning to calm the mind and body is extremely important in relieving stress. Among the easiest methods to learn are relaxation exercises. The goal of relaxation techniques is to produce a physiologic response known as a *relaxation response*—a term coined by Harvard professor and cardiologist Herbert Benson in the early 1970s to describe a physiologic response that is just the opposite of the stress response. Although an individual may relax by simply sleeping, watching television, or reading a book, relaxation exercises are designed specifically to produce the relaxation response.

With the stress response, the sympathetic nervous system dominates. With the relaxation response, the parasympathetic nervous system dominates. The parasympathetic nervous system controls bodily functions such as digestion, breathing, and heart rate during periods of rest, relaxation, visualization, meditation, and sleep. Although the sympathetic nervous system is designed to protect against immediate danger, the parasympathetic system is designed for repair, maintenance, and restoration of the body. As it relates to body weight, it can be stated that stress promotes weight gain while relaxation promotes weight loss.

THE STRESS RESPONSE VERSUS THE RELAXATION RESPONSE

THE STRESS RESPONSE

- The heart rate and force of contraction of the heart increase to provide blood to areas necessary for response to the stressor.
- Blood is shunted away from the skin and internal organs except the heart and lungs, while the amount of blood supplying required oxygen and glucose to the muscles and brain is increased.
- The rate of breathing rises to supply necessary oxygen to the heart, brain, and exercising muscle.
- Sweat production increases to eliminate toxic compounds produced by the body, and to lower body temperature.
- Production of digestive secretions is severely reduced because digestive activity is not critical to counteracting stress.
- Blood sugar levels are raised dramatically as the liver dumps stored glucose into the bloodstream.

THE RELAXATION RESPONSE

- The heart rate is reduced and the heart beats more effectively. Blood pressure is reduced.
- Blood is shunted towards internal organs, especially those organs involved in digestion.
- The rate of breathing decreases as oxygen demand is reduced during periods of rest.
- Sweat production diminishes, because a person who is calm and relaxed does not experience nervous perspiration.
- Production of digestive secretions is increased, greatly improving digestion.
- Blood sugar levels are maintained in the normal physiologic range.

Achieving the Relaxation Response

The relaxation response can be achieved through a variety of techniques. The most popular are meditation, prayer, progressive relaxation, self-hypnosis, and biofeedback. All of these techniques have the same physiologic effect: a state of deep relaxation.

One of the most popular techniques for producing the relaxation response is diaphragmatic breathing. To produce the desired long-term health benefits, set aside at least five to ten minutes each day to perform this relaxation exercise:

1. Find a comfortable and quiet place to lie down or sit.
2. Place your feet slightly apart. Place one hand on your abdomen near your navel. Place the other hand on your chest.
3. You will be inhaling through your nose and exhaling through your mouth.
4. Concentrate on your breathing. Note which hand is rising and falling with each breath.
5. Gently exhale most of the air out of your lungs.
6. Inhale while slowly counting to four. As you inhale, slightly extend your abdomen, causing it to rise about one inch. Make sure that you are not moving your chest or shoulders.
7. As you breathe in, imagine the warmed air flowing in. Imagine this warmth flowing to all parts of your body.
8. Pause for one second, then slowly exhale to a count of four. As you exhale, your abdomen should move inward.
9. As the air flows out, imagine all your tension and stress leaving your body.
10. Repeat the process until a sense of deep relaxation is achieved.

L-Theanine Promotes the Relaxation Response

L-theanine is a unique amino acid found almost exclusively in tea plants (*Camellia sinensis*). In fact, L-theanine is the primary amino acid component of green tea, comprising between 1 and 2 percent of the dry weight of tea leaves. The effects of L-theanine are truly amazing. Clinical studies have demonstrated that L-theanine reduces stress, improves the quality of sleep, diminishes the symptoms of premenstrual syndrome, heightens mental acuity, and reduces negative side effects of caffeine. These clinical effects are directly related to L-theanine's ability to stimulate the production of alpha brain waves (a state often achieved by meditation and characterized by being relaxed with greater mental focus and mental alertness) as well as to reduce beta brain waves, which are associated with nervousness, scattered thoughts, and hyper-activity.

L-theanine has been approved for use in Japan as an aid to con-quer stress and promote relaxation. It is a very popular ingredient in functional foods and beverages as well as dietary supplements de-signed to produce mental and physical relaxation without inducing drowsiness. L-theanine is fast acting. Generally, the effects are felt within the first thirty minutes, and have been shown to last up to eight to twelve hours.

Based on the results of clinical studies, it has been established that L-theanine is effective in the range of 50 to 300mg. If you have higher levels of stress, take at least 100 to 300mg one to three times daily. Al-though L-theanine is completely safe and without any known adverse drug interactions, as a general guideline it is recommended to take no more than 600mg within a six-hour period and no more than 1,200mg within a twenty-four-hour period.

L-THEANINE FOR STRESS-INDUCED EATING

Do you eat when you're under stress? L-theanine can help to control the stress-induced food cravings that lead to excess weight gain. Daily stresses and problematic sleep patterns can cause too much cortisol to surge through the body, leading to excess insulin produc-tion and weight gain. Normally, the body releases high amounts of cortisol early in the morning and only low levels at night. However, if you are under stress, your adrenals will release cortisol whenever it seems to be needed. Constant stress can cause excessive levels of cor-tisol and adrenal hormones in the body. Continuously elevated corti-

(continued on next page)

sol levels are associated with weight gain, problems with relaxation, increased sugar or carbohydrate cravings, fatigue, and a compulsion to eat. L-theanine can counteract these effects of cortisol by enhancing a feeling of calm and relaxation, thereby controlling food cravings. For best results, we recommend using L-theanine chewable tablets for a more immediate effect. Crave-Relax from Natural Factors provides 100mg of L-theanine per chewable tablet and has been used successfully in our weight-loss community programs.

LIFESTYLE FACTORS

Your lifestyle is a major determinant of your stress levels. In addition to negative coping patterns used ineffectively to diffuse stress, and failure to employ techniques that promote the relaxation response, the other primary lifestyle issues that greatly reduce a person's ability to deal with stress are poor time management, relationship issues, lack of physical exercise, and poor sleeping habits.

Time Management

Most people who are really stressed out feel that they simply do not have enough time. Here are some simple but highly effective tips for better time management:

- Set priorities. Realize that you can only accomplish so much in a day. Decide what is important, and limit your efforts to that goal.
- Organize your day. There are always interruptions and unplanned demands on your time, but create a definite plan for the day on the basis of your priorities. Avoid the pitfall of always letting the "immediate demands" control your life.
- Delegate authority. Delegate as much authority and work as you can. You can't do everything yourself. Learn to train and depend on others.
- Tackle tough jobs first. Handle the most important tasks first,

while your energy levels are high. Leave the busy work or running around for later in the day.

- Be prepared for meetings. Meetings can chew up a lot of time. A few minutes of preparation can go a long way in reducing the length of meeting times. Make sure there is a stated objective for the meeting, an organized agenda, and a timeline.

- Avoid putting things off. Work done under the pressure of an unreasonable deadline often has to be redone. That creates more stress than if it had been done right the first time. Plan ahead.

- Don't be a perfectionist. You can never really achieve perfection anyway. Do your best in a reasonable amount of time, then move on to other important tasks. If you find time, you can always come back later and polish the task some more.

Personal Relationships

It is beyond the scope of this book to provide much advice on improving your personal relationships, so let us focus on just one important area: communication. The quality of any relationship ultimately comes down to the quality of the communication. Learning to communicate effectively goes a very long way in reducing the stress and occasional (or frequent) conflicts of interpersonal relationships. Regardless of the type of personal relationship, here are seven tips for effective communication:

- Learn to be a good listener. Allow the person you are communicating with to share their feelings and thoughts uninterrupted. Emphathize with the person, put yourself in their shoes. If you first seek to understand, you will find yourself being better understood.

- Be an active listener. This means that you must be truly interested in what the other person is communicating. Listen to what they are saying instead of thinking about your response. Ask questions to gain more information or clarify what they are telling you. Good questions open lines of communication.

- Be a reflective listener. Restate or reflect back to the other person your interpretation of what they are telling you. This simple technique shows the other person that you are both listening to and understanding what they are saying. Restating what you think is being said may cause some short-term conflict in some situations, but it is certainly worth the risk.

- Wait to speak until the person you want to communicate with is listening. If the person is not ready to listen, your message will not be heard no matter how well you communicate.

- Don't try to talk over somebody. If you find yourself being interrupted, relax; don't try to out-talk the other person. If you are courteous and allow them to speak, eventually (unless extremely rude) they will respond likewise. If that doesn't happen, point out that the other person is interrupting the communication process. You can do this only if you have been a good listener. Double standards in relationships seldom work.

- Help the other person become an active listener. This can be done by asking whether they have understood what you were communicating. Ask them to tell you what they heard. If the other person doesn't seem to understand what you are saying, keep trying until they do.

- Don't be afraid of long silences. Human communication involves much more than human words. A great deal can be communicated during silences; unfortunately, in many situations silence can make us feel uncomfortable. Relax. Some people need silence to collect their thoughts and feel safe in communicating. The important thing to remember during silences is that you must remain an active listener.

Physical Exercise

The immediate effect of exercise is stress on the body. However, with a regular exercise program the body adapts, and exercise becomes an effective stress-reduction technique. With regular exercise, the body becomes stronger, functions more efficiently, and has greater endurance. Exercise is a vital component of a comprehensive stress management program, effective weight loss, and overall good health.

People who exercise regularly are much less likely to suffer from fatigue, tension, depression, feelings of inadequacy, and worries. Exercise alone has been demonstrated to have a tremendous effect in terms of improving mood and the ability to handle stressful life situations.

We discuss the importance of exercise more extensively in chapter 7, Tone Your Muscles, Train Your Heart.

SLEEP AND WEIGHT GAIN

Sleep deprivation increases hunger and slows down metabolism, making it more difficult to maintain or lose weight. It does so by:

- Increasing the level of cortisol, thereby promoting increased appetite, cravings for sugar, and weight gain. An elevated cortisol level also interferes with proper utilization of carbohydrates, leading to an increase in the storage of body fat and insulin resistance, a critical step in the development of obesity and diabetes.
- Elevating ghrelin and reducing leptin. Ghrelin is an appetite-stimulating hormone released mostly by the stomach. When ghrelin levels are up, people feel hungry. Leptin is a hormone released by fat cells that promotes a feeling of satiety.

A study conducted at the Sleep, Chronobiology, and Neuroendocrinology Research Laboratory at the University of Chicago Hospitals examined the effect of sleep deprivation on ghrelin and leptin in subjects who were limited to four hours in bed for two consecutive nights and compared them to levels measured when the subjects were allowed up to ten hours in bed for two nights. Leptin levels were 18 percent lower and ghrelin levels were 28 percent higher when the subjects only slept four hours compared to ten. In addition, the sleep-deprived men who had the biggest hormonal changes also said they felt the most hungry and craved carbohydrate-rich foods, including cakes, candy, ice cream, pasta, and bread. Those who had the smallest changes reported being the least hungry.

Getting a Good Night's Sleep

Over the course of a year, over one half of the U.S. population will have difficulty falling asleep. About 33 percent of the population experiences insomnia on a regular basis. Many use over-the-counter sedative medications to combat insomnia, while others seek stronger drugs. Insomnia can have many causes, but the most common are depression, anxiety, and tension. If psychological factors do not seem to be the cause, caffeine and medications may be responsible. In fact, well over 300 drugs have been identified that can interfere with normal sleep.

COMMON CAUSES OF INSOMNIA

Anxiety or tension	Phobia of sleep
Lack of exercise	Hypoglycemia
Depression	Disruptive environment
Environmental change	Pain or discomfort
Emotional arousal	Caffeine
Fear of insomnia	Drugs
Fear of sleep	Alcohol

Elimination of Inhibitors of Sleep

Coffee, as well as less obvious caffeine sources such as soft drinks, chocolate, coffee-flavored ice cream, hot cocoa, and tea must all be eliminated in people who suffer from insomnia. Even small amounts of caffeine such as those found in decaffeinated coffee or chocolate may be enough to cause insomnia in some people.

Alcohol must also be eliminated in people with regular insomnia. Alcohol causes the release of adrenaline and disrupts the production of serotonin (an important brain chemical that initiates sleep). Although not considered stimulants, sugar and refined carbohydrates can interfere with sleep. Eating a diet high in sugar and refined carbohydrates and eating irregularly can cause a reaction in the body that triggers the fight-or-flight response, causing wakefulness. Other food compounds that can act as stimulants include some food colorings. Adverse food reactions such as food sensitivities and allergies can also cause insomnia.

In sleep maintenance insomnia, we have found nocturnal hypoglycemia (low nighttime blood glucose level) to be a major factor. When there is a drop in the blood glucose level, it causes the release of hormones that regulate glucose levels, such as adrenaline, cortisol, glucagon, and growth hormone. These compounds stimulate the brain. They are a natural signal that it is time to eat.

The first step in eliminating sleep maintenance insomnia is stabilizing daytime and nighttime blood sugar levels. In our experience, when people get off the blood sugar roller coaster their sleep quality increases dramatically. Good bedtime snacks to keep blood sugar levels steady throughout the night are oatmeal and other whole-grain cereals taken with 2.5 to 5 grams of PGX. This dietary prescription will not only help maintain blood sugar levels; it will actually help to promote sleep by increasing the level of serotonin within the brain. Following the recommendations given in chapter 4 go a long way in promoting a good night's sleep.

Finally, foods high in tryptophan, such as turkey, milk, cottage cheese, chicken, eggs, and nuts, especially almonds, may also help to promote sleep.

EIGHT TIPS FOR PREPARING FOR A GOOD NIGHT'S SLEEP

1. **Make your bedroom primarily a place for sleeping.** It is not a good idea to use your bed for paying bills, doing work, etc. Help your body recognize that this is a place for rest or intimacy. Make sure your room is well ventilated and the temperature consistent. And try to keep it quiet. You could use a fan or a "white noise" machine to help block outside noises.

2. **Incorporate bedtime rituals.** Listening to soft music or sipping a cup of herbal tea cues your body that it's time to slow down and begin to prepare for sleep.

3. **Keep a regular schedule.** Try to go to bed and wake up at the same time every day, even on the weekends. Keeping a regular schedule will help your body expect sleep at the same time each day. Don't oversleep to make up for a poor night's sleep—doing that for even a couple of days can reset your body clock and make it hard for you to get to sleep at night.

(continued on next page)

4. **Relax for a while before going to bed.** Spending quiet time can make falling asleep easier. This may include meditation, relaxation and/or breathing exercises, or taking a warm bath. Try listening to recorded relaxation or guided imagery programs.

5. **Get out of bed if unable to sleep.** Don't lie in bed awake. Go into another room and do something relaxing until you feel sleepy. Worrying about falling asleep actually keeps many people awake.

6. **Don't do anything stimulating.** Don't read anything job-related or watch a stimulating TV program (commercials and news shows tend to be alerting). Don't expose yourself to bright light. The light gives cues to your brain that it is time to wake up.

7. **Consider changing your bedtime.** If you are experiencing sleeplessness or insomnia consistently, think about going to bed later so that the time you spend in bed is spent sleeping. If you are only getting five hours of sleep at night, figure out what time you need to get up and subract five hours (for example, if you want to get up at 6:00 a.m. go to bed at 1:00 a.m.). This may seem counterproductive and, at first, you may be depriving yourself of some sleep, but it can help train your body to sleep consistently while in bed. When you are spending all of your time in bed sleeping, you can gradually sleep more by adding fifteen minutes per night.

8. **Perform Progressive Relaxation.** This technique is based on a very simple procedure of comparing tension against relaxation. Begin with contracting the muscles of the face and neck, hold the contraction for a period of at least one to two seconds, and then relax the muscles. Next the upper arms and chest are contracted then relaxed, followed by the lower arms and hands. Repeat the process progressively down the body, i.e., the abdomen, the buttocks, the thighs, the calves, and the feet. Then work your way back up to your head. Repeat two or three times. This technique is often used in the treatment of anxiety and insomnia.

Special Dietary Supplements That Promote a Good Night's Sleep

There are a number of natural products that we have found to be extremely reliable in helping to improve sleep quality. For example, melatonin is an important hormone secreted by the pineal gland, a small gland in the center of the brain. A melatonin supplement is one of the best aids for sleep. However, it appears that the sleep-promoting effects of melatonin are most apparent only if a person's melatonin levels are low. In other words, taking melatonin is not like taking a sleeping pill. It will only produce a sedative effect when natural melatonin levels are diminished. A dosage of 3mg at bedtime is more than enough. We prefer products that are sublingual (under the tongue) or chewable tablets.

Previously, we described the effects of 5-HTP and L-theanine. Both of these compounds improve sleep quality. In particular, 5-HTP has also been shown in several double-blind clinical studies to decrease the time required to get to sleep and to decrease the number of nighttime awakenings. The recommended dosage is 50 to 100mg at bedtime.

L-theanine is also an important supplement when trying to get a better night's sleep. At typical dosages (100 to 300mg), L-theanine does not act as a sedative, but it does significantly improve sleep quality. It is also an excellent support agent to melatonin and 5-HTP at this dosage. Higher single dosages of 400 to 600mg do exert sedative action.

CHAPTER SUMMARY

- The three phases of the general adaptation syndrome are: alarm, resistance, and exhaustion.
- Elevated cortisol levels are associated with increased appetite, cravings for sugar, and weight gain.
- Cortisol exerts a double whammy on fat cells in the abdomen: it stimulates their growth and it stimulates the manufacture of new abdominal fat cells.
- Cortisol also adversely affects appetite and promotes the craving of carbohydrates by lowering brain serotonin levels.

- 5-HTP can raise brain serotonin levels helping to reduce carbohydrate cravings, promote satiety, and produce effective weight loss.
- Relaxation exercises are easy-to-learn techniques that quiet the mind and promote the relaxation response.
- L-theanine is an amino acid from green tea that reduces stress, improves the quality of sleep, and reduces food cravings.
- Effective time management is a critical goal to reduce stress.
- The quality of any relationship ultimately comes down to the quality of communication. The first key to successful communication is the most important: Learn to be a good listener.
- Sleep deprivation increases hunger and slows down metabolism.
- Even small amounts of caffeine, such as those found in decaffeinated coffee or chocolate, may be enough to cause insomnia in some people.
- When people get off the blood sugar roller coaster, their sleep quality increases dramatically.
- Melatonin is one of the best aids for sleep, but it only works when natural melatonin levels are low.
- 5-HTP and L-theanine have been shown to improve sleep quality.

7

TONE YOUR MUSCLES,
TRAIN YOUR HEART

Regular physical exercise is obviously a major key to good health, but is it an effective weight-loss strategy? The answer to this question may surprise you. Research shows exercise alone is of limited value as a weight-loss strategy. In one of the latest studies in women, even substantial increases in exercise alone were not enough to produce weight loss. To lose weight, the exercise had to be coupled with a reduced intake of calories. In contrast, men were able to lose weight through increased exercise alone. This difference might be because the men were able to burn more calories in exercise than women, or it might reflect some metabolic difference in how men and women respond to exercise. We think we know the real answer to this riddle. It has to do with muscle mass. The ability to lose weight with exercise is a direct reflection of a person's muscle mass. Since men have a larger muscle mass than women, the effect of exercise alone as a weight-loss strategy is more apparent in men.

The more muscle mass that you have, the more fat you burn. Muscle mass is the primary fat-burning furnace in the body. A muscle cell burns as much as fifteen times more calories per day than a fat cell. The importance of building muscle mass for effective weight loss cannot be overstated. Likewise, muscle mass is the primary factor that will determine how quickly you can lose weight even if you are carefully following a sensible weight-loss plan. Low muscle mass is a primary reason why many people hit a plateau at some point during a weight-loss program.

For these reasons, radical diets that result in significant loss of muscle need to be avoided at all costs. They may work in the short run, but they set you up for failure later on. Instead, it is vital that you follow a plan that avoids loss of muscle while you lose weight. The Hunger Free Forever program has been shown to preserve muscle mass while you lose weight. Most of our patients increase their lean muscle mass and end up with no decrease (in fact, often an increase) in their resting metabolic rate at the end of the program. The fact is that increasing your muscle mass is one of the best ways to ensure that you can keep your weight off over the long haul without having to endure hunger or feel deprived of the joy of eating.

In this chapter, we are going to stress the general importance of exercise in a weight-loss program with our own prescription for the best types of exercise for maximum benefit. But first, we want to introduce to you the little-known term sarcopenia. It comes from the Greek meaning "poverty of flesh." Sarcopenia is the degenerative loss of skeletal muscle mass and strength as we age. It is to our muscle mass what osteoporosis is to our bones. The combination of osteoporosis and sarcopenia results in the significant frailty often seen in the elderly population. The degree of sarcopenia as we age is a predictor of disability and is linked to decreased vitality, poor balance, slower gait speed, falls, and fractures.

As in the prevention of osteoporosis where we want to build our bones while we are young to help us preserve them longer through the aging process, the same is true for sarcopenia. We want to build our muscle mass now to prevent premature aging. As it is important to engage in dietary, lifestyle, and exercise strategies to ward off osteoporosis in our later years, we must do the same to ward off sarcopenia.

SARCOPENIA: CAUSES AND SOLUTIONS

Because of higher levels of testosterone and activities that favor the growth of muscle, men usually start their adult lives with more muscle mass than women, and often an appetite to match their raging metabolism. In both men and women, muscle mass increases throughout adolescence and peaks during the late teens through the mid- to late twenties. After that, muscle mass declines slowly, but quite relentlessly, in most people. In fact, unless muscles are specifically exercised through weight training, we lose about 1 percent of our lean muscle mass every year until we are 50. In our fifties the rate of decline is slightly accelerated, but the real decline begins at age 60. By the time we reach the age of 80 our muscle mass is often less than half of what it was in our twenties. What causes this loss in muscle mass? Of course a lack of muscle-specific exercise is primarily to blame. However, we also know that muscle cells lose their ability to respond to growthpromoting substances—especially insulin and insulin-like growth factors—as we age, particularly as we gain weight. We see once again the importance of increasing the sensitivity of our cells to the hormone insulin. In reality, in early adulthood, we don't even know we are accumulating fat because as we gain fat we also lose muscle and our weight may be relatively stable or it may not increase as much as the weight of fat we are depositing. By the time we are in our fifties or sixties we may not be seriously overweight, but we may have very low lean muscle mass.

Another key factor in the development of sarcopenia is inflammation, not the kind of fiery inflammation that occurs when you sprain your ankle or scrape your knee, but the type of inflammation that is emerging as the underlying feature in virtually every chronic degenerative disease including heart disease, cancer, stroke, diabetes, and Alzheimer's disease. In fact, this kind of inflammation is a close partner to insulin resistance and is a direct result of substances released from excessive internal belly fat.

C-Reactive Protein

Silent inflammation is an important factor in the development of sarcopenia. To measure the degree of inflammation, physicians can determine the level of C-reactive protein (CRP) in the blood. CRP is one of the acute phase proteins that increase during the systemic inflammation that often accompanies insulin resistance. Most of the research on CRP has focused on its role in predicting heart attack. The higher the CRP level, the higher the risk of developing heart attack. The same is true for sarcopenia: the higher the CRP level, the greater the acceleration in the loss of muscle mass. Elevated CRP levels are also associated with a significantly higher risk for the development of insulin resistance and type 2 diabetes.

We recommend that part of your annual physical exam include blood work (see page 41) to determine your CRP levels. The goal is to keep your CRP level below 1.0mg/L. At this level, there is little silent inflammation occurring. If your CRP is between 1.0 and 3.0mg/L, that is a major caution. If your CRP is higher than 3.0mg/L, it is a serious red flag.

Dietary interventions alone have been shown to lower CRP levels. In particular, the Mediterranean diet can be quite effective in lowering CRP levels to normal. If you follow its basic dietary recommendations, your CRP level should easily fall into the normal range. In addition, recent population-based studies have shown carotene-rich foods are protective against a decline in muscle strength and walking disability as we get older. Good sources of carotenes include dark-colored vegetables such as carrots, squash, spinach, kale, tomatoes, yams, and sweet potatoes; and fruits such as tomatoes, cantaloupe, watermelon, apricots, and citrus.

THE MEDITERRANEAN DIET

The traditional Mediterranean diet provides significant protection against silent inflammation. However, it does not mean you should eat more Italian restaurant food. The Mediterranean diet reflects food patterns in the early 1960s typical of Crete, parts of the rest of Greece, and southern Italy. This diet has shown tremendous benefit in fighting heart disease and cancer, as well as diabetes. It centers on most of the principles of the Hunger Free Forever program, specifically:

• An abundance of plant food, including fruit, legumes, and vegetables

• Breads, pasta, potatoes, nuts, and seeds eaten regularly and in modest portions

• Minimally processed foods with a focus on seasonal, fresh, and locally grown foods

- Fresh fruit daily, with sweets containing concentrated sugars or honey consumed a few times per week at most
- Low-fat dairy products, principally cheese and yogurt, consumed daily in low to moderate amounts
- Fresh fish consumed on almost a daily basis
- Poultry and eggs consumed in moderate amounts, about one to four times weekly, or not at all
- Red meat consumed in small, infrequent amounts
- Olive oil as the principal source of fat
- Wine consumed in low to moderate amounts, normally with meals.

The traditional Mediterranean diet was a high-satiety way of eating that emphasized eating low caloric–density foods in abundance while limiting portions of higher calorie foods. Every meal was a celebration of family and friends, where food was eaten slowly and mindfully, and people savored every bite. Moderation was an esteemed virtue, and obesity rates were traditionally low.

Strength Training Reduces Sarcopenia

The most important step to preventing sarcopenia is to follow a regular strength-training program by lifting weights or engaging in resistance exercises. The benefits of strength training are vast, particularly for women and for people over age 50. In addition to helping burn more fat, a larger muscle mass is associated with a healthier heart, improved joint function, relief from arthritis pain, better antioxidant protection, and higher self-esteem. We have found that many women do not strength train because they fear gaining weight, but just the opposite occurs. Building muscle mass actually helps to burn calories more effectively.

You don't have to lift barbells or utilize clumsy machines to strength train. Resistance exercises include those that utilize your body weight. There are even forms of yoga that help to build strength and muscle mass. We provide an exercise routine that you can do at home with no exercise equipment later on in this chapter.

Many of our women patients have found Curves to be an excellent introduction to strength training. Curves uses hydraulic resistance equipment rather than weights. This is easier on the tendons and ligaments for people who have not been involved previously in regular weight training. Their program also gets you to move from one station to another over a short period of time, so your heart rate stays elevated for the entire workout. (This is called circuit training.) In this way, you enjoy the benefits of increased muscle mass as well as cardiovascular fitness in the same workout. The disadvantage to Curves is that it is not available to men. However, circuit training can be easily carried out at any gym with some basic instruction. It can usually be done safely three times per week or even more often if the intensity is not too high.

For women and men who want to see greater increases in muscle mass from strength training, more conventional weight training using heavier weights and more concentrated exercises is preferred over Curves-style workouts. One or two intensive weight workouts per week can provide significant increases in lean muscle, and aerobic exercise can be carried out on other days.

The Importance of Protein

Along with its satiety-promoting properties, dietary protein is essential in supporting muscle growth and fighting sarcopenia. If you want to gain control over your weight, consuming adequate amounts of protein throughout the day is vital. In the Hunger Free Forever program, we make sure our patients understand that they need adequate amounts of protein with every meal they eat, including breakfast. Lean meats, legumes, and low-fat dairy products should be consumed with most meals.

Protein supplements can be used to balance out any meal that is low in protein or when you are preparing a smoothie as a meal. The best choice for protein supplementation is whey protein. Whey protein is a natural by-product of the cheesemaking process. Cow's milk has about 6.25 percent protein. Of that protein, 80 percent is casein (another type of protein) and the remaining 20 percent is whey. When cheese is made, it uses the casein molecules, leaving whey. Whey protein is made by filtering off the other components of whey such as lactose, fats, and minerals. Whey protein is easier to digest and is better tolerated than casein. Even those who are dairy intolerant usually have no difficulties with a high-quality whey protein isolate or concentrate.

Whey protein has the highest biological value of all proteins. Biological value is used to rate protein based on how much of the protein consumed is actually absorbed, retained, and used in the body. One of the key reasons why the biological value of whey protein is so high is that it has the highest concentrations of glutamine and branched chain amino acids (BCAAs) found in nature. These amino acids are critical to cellular health, muscle growth, and protein synthesis.

Although the most popular use of whey protein is by body builders and athletes looking to increase their protein intake, whey protein is also used to support recovery from surgery, prevent the "wasting syndrome" of AIDS, and offset some of the negative effects of radiation therapy and chemotherapy. Whey protein use is also particularly important in battling sarcopenia. It has also been demonstrated in clinical trials (compared to a placebo) to produce greater strength and muscle mass gains in elderly subjects involved in weight-training programs.

You can find whey protein powder in a variety of flavors, including vanilla, chocolate, and strawberry, in premeasured individual serving packets and bulk canisters in the "body building" section of a health-food store. In our clinical research center, we recommend high-quality whey protein concentrates or isolates for smoothies, and utilize whey protein within the SlimStyles meal replacement formulas with PGX from Natural Factors.

The total protein requirement for long-term weight maintenance in adults is about 0.4g per pound of body weight per day. If you are actively building muscle, you should be aiming for 0.6 to 0.9g per pound of body weight per day. The most convenient and cost-effective way to do this is by using high-protein meal replacement beverages and adding whey protein to low-calorie smoothies. In most cases, our patients will consume 25 to 50 grams of supplemental protein from whey or from whey-based meal replacements throughout the day.

Creatine

Creatine is one of the most popular nutritional supplements for athletes and bodybuilders. It is used primarily to increase strength and lean body mass and has shown consistent results in promoting these effects in clinical studies. Creatine is used in muscle tissue for the production of phosphocreatine, an important factor in the formation of ATP, the source of energy for muscle contraction and many other functions in the body. Creatine supplementation works by increasing phosphocreatine levels in muscle and improving muscle protein synthesis, letting you work just a bit harder during your strength-training workout sessions.

Creatine supplementation appears to be useful in battling sarcopenia, but it must be combined with weight training. When combined with weight training, creatine supplementation has been shown to increase muscle mass and improve leg strength, endurance, and power in both elderly and younger subjects. Creatine supplementation augments the muscle growth stimulation of weight training, but without the weight training it has little, if any, benefit. Our dosage recommendation is based upon body weight. Take 1 gram of creatine for every 50 pounds of body weight before you work out. If you weigh 150 pounds your dosage would be 3 grams. If you suffer from any kidney or liver disease, please consult a physician before supplementing with creatine.

A COMPREHENSIVE NUTRITIONAL APPROACH TO PREVENT SARCOPENIA

- Reduce the amount of saturated fat, trans fatty acids, cholesterol, and total fat in your diet by eating only lean sources of protein and more plant foods.
- Increase your intake of omega-3 oils by eating flaxseed oil, walnuts, and cold-water fish such as salmon. Eat at least two, but no more than three, servings of fish per week.
- Increase your intake of monounsaturated fats and the amino acid arginine by eating regular but moderate amounts of nuts and seeds

tion, and helps your body to set a lowered programmed weight. Other reasons to exercise when you are trying to lose weight are:

- When weight loss is achieved by dieting without exercise, a substantial portion of the total weight loss comes from the lean tissue, primarily as water loss.
- When exercise is included in a weight-loss program, there is usually an improvement in body composition due to a gain in lean body weight because of an increase in muscle mass and an accompanying decrease in body fat.
- Exercise increases the basal metabolic rate for an extended period of time following the exercise session. Thus extra calories are consumed for many hours after each exercise session.
- Moderate to intense exercise may have an appetite suppressant effect.
- Individuals who exercise during and after weight reduction are better able to maintain the weight loss than those who do not exercise.
- Exercise helps diminish anxiety and reduces depression, two major factors that drive people to the refrigerator in their search to find a sense of comfort.

While the immediate effect of exercise is stress on the body, with regular exercise the body adapts; it becomes stronger, functions more efficiently, and has greater endurance. The entire body benefits from regular exercise, largely as a result of improved cardiovascular and respiratory function. Exercise enhances the transport of oxygen and nutrients into cells. At the same time, exercise enhances the transport of carbon dioxide and waste products from the tissues of the body to the bloodstream and ultimately to the eliminative organs. As a result, regular exercise increases stamina and energy levels.

Diet, Exercise, and the National Weight Control Registry

Several years ago researchers James Hill, Ph.D. and Rena Wing, Ph.D. from the University of Colorado and Brown University, respectively,

such as almonds, Brazil nuts, coconut, hazelnuts, macadamia
pecans, pine nuts, pistachios, and sesame and sunflower seeds
by using a monounsaturated oil such as olive, macadami
canola for cooking purposes.

- Eat five or more servings daily of a combination of vegetable
  fruits, especially green, orange, and yellow vegetables, darl
  ored berries, and citrus fruits.

- Limit your intake of refined carbohydrates. Sugar and other r
  carbohydrates lead to the development of insulin resistance, v
  in turn, is associated with increased silent inflammation, the
  of sarcopenia.

- Utilize the benefits of whey protein by taking 25 to 50 gr
  whey protein daily.

- If you are on a strength-training program, take 1 gram of c
  for every 50 pounds of body weight before you work out.

EXERCISE AND WEIC

Regular physical exercise is obviously a vital key to good healtl
know this fact, yet only a small fraction—less than 20 per
Americans exercise on a regular basis. Physical inactivity is
reason why so many Americans are overweight. This statemen
cially true in children, as studies have demonstrated that cl
obesity is associated more with inactivity than overeating. St
dence suggests that more than 86 percent of adult obesity |
childhood. It could thus be concluded that lack of physical :
the major cause of obesity in America today.

If you are trying to lose weight, you definitely need to e
well. When you cut back on your caloric intake, it lowers y
metabolic rate (BMR)—in other words, your body slows dow
pensate. Sometimes the reduction in BMR is equal to the deg
orie deficit, so it keeps your weight basically the same. Ex
been shown to compensate for a reduced BMR due to calor

A NEAT WAY TO EXERCISE

Mayo Clinic researchers have discovered that long-term weight control may be easier to maintain by focusing less on exercise and more on increasing non-exercise energy expenditure, also referred to as non-exercise activity thermogenesis or NEAT. Examples of NEAT activities include the maintenance of posture, activities of daily living, and even fidgeting. For example, a person of normal weight typically burns 350 more calories per day from the collective impact of numerous small activities and movements. Burning 350 calories per day is equivalent to about 40 pounds of fat in one year so this may be a very important factor in long-term weight control. We provide examples of how to increase NEAT activities in chapter 8.

decided to study the secrets of success in those who lost weight and had been able to keep it off. People who had lost at least 30 pounds and had kept it off for at least one year were interviewed and placed in a database known as the National Weight Loss Registry. Over 5,000 participants have now been studied and some interesting facts have been uncovered. On average, this group has lost 66 pounds and has kept it off for five and a half years. The researchers noted that there were a wide variety of diets or programs that these successful people used to lose their weight, but exercise was the one thing that most of them had in common. In fact, 89 percent of registry participants used both diet and physical activity to lose weight, only 10 percent used diet alone, and 1 percent used exercise alone.

They shared some common behaviors in maintaining their weight loss as well. Most of the participants reported eating a relatively low-fat diet and nearly all reported eating breakfast almost every day. They also weigh themselves regularly and have a plan if their weight hits a certain maximum point. Finally, the majority of these successful long-term "losers" engage in high levels of physical activity for at least an hour every day. The lesson to be learned from this landmark study? No matter what the tabloid ads tell you, diet and exercise are both essential if you want to enjoy long-term weight control!

THE BENEFITS OF REGULAR EXERCISE

MUSCULOSKELETAL SYSTEM

Increases muscle strength and muscle mass

Increases flexibility of muscles and range of joint motion

Produces stronger bones, ligaments, and tendons

Lessens chance of injury

Enhances posture, poise, and physique

Prevents osteoporosis

HEART AND BLOOD VESSELS

Lowers resting heart rate

Strengthens heart function

Lowers blood pressure

Improves oxygen delivery throughout the body

Increases blood supply to muscles

Enlarges the arteries that provide blood to the heart muscle

Reduces the risk of coronary heart disease

Helps lower blood cholesterol and triglyceride levels

Raises levels of HDL, the "good" cholesterol

BODILY PROCESSES

Improves immune function

Aids digestion and elimination

Increases endurance and energy levels

Increases insulin sensitivity

Promotes lean body mass; burns fat

Improves sexual function in both men and women

MENTAL PROCESSES

Provides a natural release from pent-up feelings

Helps reduce tension and anxiety

Improves mental outlook and self-esteem

Helps relieve moderate depression

Improves the ability to handle stress

Stimulates improved mental function

Induces relaxation and improves sleep

The Best Exercises for Maximum Benefit

We recommend a combination of aerobic, strength-training, and flexibility exercises. Aerobic exercise refers to movement that increases utilization of oxygen. Aerobic exercises include walking briskly, jogging, bicycling, cross-country skiing, swimming, aerobic dance, and racquet sports. Strength-training (anaerobic) exercises include lifting weights and other resistance exercises as well as certain types of yoga. Circuit training, like the program at Curves, involves lighter resistance and higher repetitions of each exercise done with little rest between sets. Circuit training has some muscle-building benefits, along with greater aerobic or cardiovascular benefits than conventional weight training. We believe that there is too much focus on aerobic exercises for weight loss, and that strength-training exercise is actually more critical to long-term weight control, because it is able to build muscle mass. For overall health and fitness, we recommend engaging in both, as well as performing regular stretching exercises to maintain flexibility. Yoga, tai chi, and stretching classes are fantastic ways to increase flexibility.

AEROBIC EXERCISE VERSUS STRENGTH TRAINING FOR WEIGHT LOSS

AEROBIC EXERCISE GENERALLY
- Burns more calories per hour than weight training.
- Builds little muscle.
- Has minimal effects on metabolism in the hours after exercise.
- Has greater effects on metabolism when workout is very hard.
- Can be done every day.
- Needs to be done at least three times per week for sustained benefits.

WEIGHT TRAINING
- Raises resting basal metabolic rate (BMR).
- Raises the metabolism for several hours after the workout.
- Should be limited to three or four times per week.
- Produces benefits from as little as one hard workout per week.

If you are not currently exercising, we recommend walking. Brisk walking is a great activity because it works the muscles of the lower body, the largest muscles in the body. If you are going to walk on a regular basis, we strongly urge you to first purchase a pair of high-quality walking or jogging shoes to avoid foot and ankle issues.

Walking is more enjoyable if you make it a social event. Locate one or two people in your neighborhood with whom you would enjoy walking. If you are meeting one or two people, you will certainly be more regular than if you depend solely on your own intentions. Commit to walking three to five mornings or afternoons each week. Increase the exercise duration from an initial ten minutes to at least thirty minutes.

Once you have reached thirty minutes of brisk walking, and can do this comfortably, then increase your pace. You can do this by walking for five minutes, then breaking into a slow trot for five minutes, and then alternating walking and slow trotting for thirty minutes. This will obviously increase the distance you cover, as well as the amount of exercise. You can also increase the intensity of this exercise by gradually increasing the amount of time you jog.

For strength training, if you do not want to join a health club and have limited access to exercise equipment, here is a set of at-home exercises that can be used instead. Do fifteen repetitions with each exercise and cycle through each exercise three times for a complete workout.

At-home resistance exercise program

1. Squats
- Place your feet about shoulder-width apart.
- Keeping your upper body straight and tall, bend your knees as far down as you feel comfortable when first starting out, but try to get your thighs parallel to the ground. Lower to a count of four.
- Using leg power, slowly push yourself back up to the start position to a count of two.

2. Chest
- Stand facing a wall, about 2 feet from it, with your feet hips-width apart.
- Place your hands on the wall just outside shoulder-width apart.
- Bending only at the elbows, lower yourself forward towards the wall to a count of four and then push back to the starting position to a count of two.
- Keep your body stiff and straight during the movement.

3. Shoulders (If you don't have dumbbells, you can use soup cans or water bottles. You don't need a lot of weight for this exercise.)
- Stand erect with your arms at your sides, holding a dumbbell in each hand.
- Keeping your arms straight, raise them palms down in front of you to shoulder height to a count of two.
- Next, extend your arms out to your sides to a count of two; then slowly, to a count of four, bring your arms straight down to your sides.

4. Biceps
- Stand with your feet hips-width apart, knees slightly bent, and arms at your sides.
- With your right hand at your side, place your left palm into your right palm.
- Apply resistance with your left hand as you slowly bring your right hand up, bending only at the elbow, to a count of two.
- Once at the top, slowly return your right hand to your side, applying resistance the whole time with your left hand, to a count of four.
- Repeat 15 times, then switch sides.

5. Triceps
- Sit on the side edge of a flat bench or the front edge of a chair.
- Place your hands on the edge of the chair beside your buttocks and grip the edge.

- Your feet should be flat on the floor, about two feet in front of you, with your knees bent.
- Lift yourself off the chair so you are now supporting yourself on your hands.
- Bend your arms, dipping your body down. Go down only as far as you feel comfortable to a count of four, being careful not to touch the chair.
- Push back up by extending your arms to a count of two.
- It is important to keep your back close to the edge of the chair as you do these to minimize shoulder stress.

6. Abdominals
- Lie down flat on your back with your knees bent and your feet on the floor.
- Cross your arms by placing the palms of your hands on the opposite shoulder.
- Perform a crunch by lifting your chest and head up towards the ceiling, pushing your lower back flat on the floor.
- Hold at the top of the movement for a second and concentrate on squeezing your abdominal muscles hard.
- Slowly lower back down and repeat.

7. Calves
- Stand on the edge of a step on only the balls of your feet.
- Keeping knees stiff and bending only at the ankles, lower your heels down towards the floor until you feel a strong stretch in your calves.
- Slowly push up as high as you can, pausing at the top and contracting the calf muscles.
- Do both legs at the same time to begin; as you get stronger, do one leg at a time.

HOW TO CREATE AN EFFECTIVE EXERCISE PROGRAM

Exercise is clearly one of the most powerful medicines available. Just imagine if all of the benefits of exercise could be put in a pill. Unfortunately, it is not that easy. The time you spend exercising is a valuable investment toward good health. To help you develop a successful exercise program, here are seven steps to follow.

Step 1. Make a Solid Commitment to Exercise

The first step is realizing just how important it is to get regular exercise. We cannot stress enough how vital regular exercise is to your health. But as much as we emphasize this fact, it means absolutely nothing unless it really sinks in and you accept it as well. You must make regular exercise a top priority in your life. If you have time to eat and sleep, you have time to exercise. It's really a matter of priorities. If exercise is important enough, you will find the time and expend the energy. Examine all of the things that keep you from exercising and find solutions to those barriers.

BARRIERS TO EXERCISE AND SOLUTIONS

One of the keys to starting and successfully keeping with an exercise program is to identify your personal barriers to exercise and then create solutions to overcome those barriers. Rather than making excuses, find a creative way to overcome these obstacles and make exercise a daily commitment.

Barriers to Exercise	Example Solutions
Injury or poor health	Aquacise, recumbent exercise bike
Child care responsibilities	Bring kids along; fitness center with child care
Lack of time	Get up a bit early; shut off the TV
Lack of money	Walk; work out at home; dance in your room to music
Lack of motivation	Walk a pet; exercise with friends
Too tired	Exercise will give you energy
Isolation	Join a walking club; go to a gym or Curves
Climate	Indoor walking tracks; home equipment

Step 2. Consult Your Physician

If you are not currently on a regular exercise program, get medical clearance if you have health problems or if you are over 40 years of age. The main concern is the functioning of your heart. Exercise can be quite harmful (and even fatal) if your heart is not able to meet the increased demands placed on it.

It is especially important to see a physician if any of the following applies to you: heart disease; smoking; high blood pressure; extreme breathlessness with physical exertion; pain or pressure in chest, arm, teeth, jaw, or neck with exercise; dizziness or fainting; abnormal heart rhythm (palpitations or irregular beat).

Step 3. Select an Activity You Can Enjoy

If you are fit enough to begin with, the next thing to do is select an activity that you would enjoy. The key to getting the maximum benefit from exercise is to make it enjoyable. Choose activities that you like and have fun with. If you can find enjoyment in exercise, you are much more likely to exercise regularly. One way to make it fun is to get a workout partner or join a workout class. Another, using the list below, is to choose from one to five of the activities, or fill in a choice or two of your own. Make a commitment to do one activity a day for at least twenty minutes and preferably an hour. Make your goal to derive pleasure from the activity.

Gardening	Jazzercise	Heavy housecleaning
Bicycling	Dancing	Yoga
Walking	Bowling	Pilates
Swimming	Stationary bike	Tai chi
Golfing	Treadmill	Skiing
Tennis	Stair climbing	Snowshoeing
Jogging	Weight lifting	

Step 4. Monitor Exercise Intensity

Exercise intensity is determined by measuring your heart rate—the number of times your heart beats per minute. This determination can be quickly done by placing your index and middle finger of one hand on the side of your neck just below the angle of the jaw or on the inside of opposite wrist. Beginning with zero, count the number of heartbeats for six seconds. Simply add a zero to this number and you have your pulse. For example, if you counted 14 beats, your heart rate would be 140. As an alternative to counting your pulse, a wireless heart rate monitor is a very worthwhile investment. Good ones can now be acquired for under $75 at any running store. For most people, the simplest models are best. Many of our patients never exercise without their wireless heart rate monitor.

A quick and easy way to determine your maximum training heart rate is simply to subtract your age from 185. For example, if you are 40 years old your maximum heart rate would be 145. To determine the bottom of the training zone, simply subtract 20 from this number. In the case of a 40-year-old this would be 125. So, the training range for a 40-year-old would be between 125 and 145 beats per minute. For maximum health benefits, you must stay in this range and never exceed it. If you have a wireless heart rate monitor, for convenience you can set it to beep if you are above or below this zone.

Step 5. Do It Often

You don't get in good physical condition by exercising once; it must be performed on a regular basis. A minimum of fifteen to twenty minutes of exercising at your training heart rate at least three times a week is necessary to gain any significant cardiovascular benefits from exercise. It is better to exercise at the lower end of your training zone for longer periods of time than it is to exercise at a higher intensity for a shorter period of time.

For weight control, you should strive to exercise for an hour on most days. Two or three weight workouts per week and three or four aerobic workouts is a good balance for most people who want to lose weight and keep it off.

Step 6. Stay Motivated

No matter how committed a person is to regular exercise, at some point in time they are going to be faced with a loss of enthusiasm for working out. Here is a suggestion: Take a break. Not a long break, but skipping just one or two workouts gives your enthusiasm and motivation a chance to recoup so that you can come back with an even stronger commitment.

Here are some other suggestions to help you to stay motivated:

- Read or thumb through fitness magazines like *Men's Fitness, Muscle & Fitness*, and *Self*. Looking at pictures of people in fantastic shape is really inspirational. In addition, these magazines typically feature articles on new exercise routines.
- Set exercise goals that can easily be achieved. Write down your daily exercise goal and check it off when you have completed it.
- Appreciate your progress. Keep a record of your activities and progress. Sometimes it is hard to see the progress you are making, but if you write in a journal you'll have a permanent record of your progress. Keeping track of your progress will motivate you to continued improvement.

Step 7: Add Variety

Variety is vital to staying interested in exercise. Many people exercise for a while and then quit because it becomes too monotonous. Doing the same thing every day also puts you at risk for overuse injuries, especially if you are very heavy or you are working out a bit too long or hard for your level of conditioning. We encourage our patients to cross train. A typical example would be two strength workouts per week, three brisk walks, one swim, and a day of rest. Another week might include a treadmill workout a couple of times per week rather than an outdoor walk, or a bike ride when the weather is really nice. Or, if you really want to spice things up, how about a week featured by entering a race/walk for a favorite charity, mountain biking, mountain climbing, and belly dancing.

CHAPTER SUMMARY

- The ability to lose weight with exercise is a direct reflection of a person's muscle mass.

- The more muscle mass you have, the more fat you burn.
- Sarcopenia is the degenerative loss of skeletal muscle mass and strength as we age.
- One of the key reasons for muscle mass loss as we age is that muscle cells lose their ability to respond to growth-promoting substances, especially insulin and insulin-like-growth factors, as we age, and particularly as we gain weight.
- Silent inflammation is an important factor in the development of sarcopenia.
- Eating the Mediterranean diet has been shown to reduce silent inflammation as evidenced by a reduction in C-reactive protein levels.
- The most important step to preventing sarcopenia is to follow a regular strength-training program.
- Dietary protein is essential in supporting muscle growth and fighting sarcopenia. The best choice for protein supplementation is whey protein.
- When combined with weight training, creatine supplementation has been shown to increase muscle mass and improve leg strength, endurance, and power in both elderly and young subjects.
- Physical inactivity is a major reason why so many Americans are overweight.
- Exercise has been shown to compensate for a reduced basal metabolic rate (BMR) due to calorie restriction.
- We recommend a combination of aerobic, strength training, and flexibility exercises to see the full benefits of exercise.
- The time you spend exercising is a valuable investment toward good health.

8

REV UP YOUR METABOLISM

Have you ever had a friend who could eat all the food she wanted and still stay thin, while sometimes it felt that if you simply looked at food it tended to go right to your hips or midsection? The explanation you have probably heard is that it is a difference in metabolism. This answer is absolutely correct. However, there is probably no concept that is more misunderstood than that of metabolism and its relationship to weight control.

Without question, metabolism plays a central role in weight loss and an even more vital role in the long-term maintenance of healthy weight. In fact, some of the most important breakthroughs in obesity research are recent discoveries related specifically to metabolism. At our clinical research center, we have been carefully examining the relationship of metabolism to weight loss and we have seen how applying principles of metabolism management can be a major factor in our patients' success.

We have been fortunate to be able to utilize high-tech equipment that allows us directly to measure both body composition and metabolism in our patients. With this technology we have been able to monitor how the Hunger Free Forever program impacts these vital parameters. We have learned that weight loss must be better than just numbers dropping on a scale. We now believe that it is vital to burn fat and avoid losing muscle. It is also critical to manage and tune metabolism so that fat doesn't just pile back on after successful weight loss. Effective, permanent weight loss requires switching the metabolism from fat storing to fat burning. A highly efficient fat-burning body is much better able to control food intake and feel satisfied with food for many reasons, but, most important, it reflects a more optimal physiology.

The Hunger Free Forever program is revolutionary because it brings about consistent weight loss while maintaining lean body mass and resting (basal) metabolic rate. Because this program works by restoring the body's sensitivity to insulin, starving muscle becomes more effectively nourished, and fat can be burned while muscle mass is maintained or often even increased.

WHERE DO ALL THE CALORIES GO?

Metabolism really refers to the breakdown of food into energy that is used for every purpose required for life. The amount of energy contained in food is expressed in terms of kilocalories, which we commonly refer to as calories. This is a measurement of heat. In reality, food is "burned" inside our cells and most of the energy is trapped to be used for thousands of bodily processes. Some of this energy is released as heat to keep our bodies warm. This is similar to the fuel in your car's engine. The fuel is burned and the energy released is mostly captured and used to propel your car. A small percentage of the energy produces heat that is mostly discharged into the environment or used to heat the inside of your car on a cold day.

Maintaining an ideal body weight has everything to do with balance. If we consume more calories than our body can burn, excess food will be stored as fat. In fact, even normal weight people store a great deal of energy that they could draw on in a famine situation. For example, a lean, 155-pound man carries about 35 pounds of fat on his body, which holds about 150,000 calories (kcal) of stored energy or enough to keep him alive during starvation for a couple of months. Most of the people we work with live in a body that is composed of more than 50 percent fat. This means, for example, that a 250-pound person who is 50 percent fat carries 125 pounds or 437,500 calories (kcal) of energy on their body as stored fat. This much fat has the potential to provide all of their energy needs for almost one year!

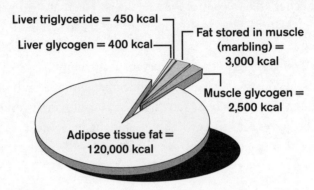

Body Energy Store of Lean 70-kg Man

Liver triglyceride = 450 kcal

Liver glycogen = 400 kcal

Fat stored in muscle (marbling) = 3,000 kcal

Muscle glycogen = 2,500 kcal

Adipose tissue fat = 120,000 kcal

Figure 8:1. Total Stored Energy in a Lean 70kg Man.

Total Energy Expenditure

Your body consumes energy in three different ways: resting energy expenditure, activity energy expenditure, and the thermic effect of food. Resting energy expenditure refers to the amount of energy your body consumes at rest. The brain, heart, liver, kidneys, and muscles consume the majority of your daily calories even while you're sleeping. Resting energy expenditure is what we typically refer to when we speak of metabolism or metabolic rate. Exercise and other daily activities consume a more variable amount of calories, depending upon your occupation, your daily activities, and your commitment to exercise. The thermic effect of food is the energy you burn in digesting food, processing nutrients, and in generating heat to warm your body.

DO OVERWEIGHT PEOPLE HAVE A SLOW METABOLISM?

The truth is that most overweight or obese people do not suffer from a low resting metabolic rate. As you gain weight, you're actually gaining mostly fat, but also some muscle. For example, cattle are sent to feed lots near the end of their lives to be overfed so that they will gain a considerable amount of well-marbled muscle. Well-marbled muscle may not be very high-quality muscle, but it still burns more energy at rest

Components of Daily Energy Expenditure

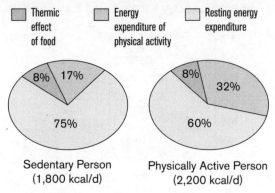

Thermic effect of food Energy expenditure of physical activity Resting energy expenditure

Sedentary Person
(1,800 kcal/d)

Physically Active Person
(2,200 kcal/d)

Segal KR et al., *Am J Clin Nutr*, 1984; 40:995–1000.

Figure 8:2. Daily Energy Expenditure in Sedentary and Active Adults.

than fat. Even fat at rest burns some calories. Numerous studies have verified that resting (basal) metabolic rate, which is the majority of calories that most people burn in a day, increases as human body weight increases. At our clinical research center, we have been able to verify that most overweight and obese people have relatively high resting metabolic rates. However, there are exceptions. In older people, especially those with very low lean body mass (sarcopenia), resting metabolic rate may be quite low even if they are heavy.

Studies have shown that rather than gaining weight due to slow metabolism, overweight or obese people often underestimate the amount of food they eat by as much as 30 percent. Careful research has shown that many people who are overweight or obese consume calories mindlessly. This is why we recommend keeping careful food records early on in weight loss and repeating your record keeping periodically. This can help you to become more mindful about your food consumption.

You can take steps to increase your resting metabolic rate. As we discussed in the last chapter, the principal way to increase your basal metabolic rate is by committing to a regular program of strength training. If you increase your lean muscle mass, you will burn extra calories

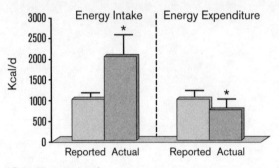

Discrepancy Between Reported and Actual Energy Intake and Expenditure

*P<0.05 vs reported

Lichtman et al., *N Engl J Med,* 1992; 327:1893.

Figure 8.3. Actual and Reported Energy Intake and Expenditure in Obese Adults.

FACTORS THAT INFLUENCE BASAL METABOLIC RATE (BMR)

Body size: Metabolic rate increases as weight, height, and surface area increase.

Body composition: Fat tissue has a lower metabolic activity than muscle tissue. As lean muscle mass increases, metabolic rate increases.

Gender: The BMR averages 5 to 10 percent lower in women than in men. This is largely because women generally possess more body fat and less muscle mass than men of similar size.

Age: A decrease in lean muscle mass during adulthood results in a slow, steady decline of roughly 0.3 percent per year in BMR after the age of about 30. This can be largely avoided by strength training throughout adulthood.

Climate and body temperature: The BMR of people in tropical climates is generally 5 to 20 percent higher than their counterparts living in more temperate areas because it takes energy to keep the body cool. Exercise performed in hot weather also imposes an additional metabolic load. Body fat content and effectiveness of clothing determine the magnitude of increase in energy metabolism in cold environments; it takes energy to keep the body warm if you work or exercise in very cold weather.

Hormonal levels: Thyroxine (T_4), the key hormone released by the thyroid glands has a significant effect upon metabolic rate. Hypothyroidism is relatively common, especially in women near or after menopause. Everyone with a weight problem should have their thyroid function checked by their doctor and treated appropriately if it turns out to be low.

Health: Fever, illness, or injury may increase resting metabolic rate two-fold.

around the clock. Improving insulin sensitivity by consuming PGX with each meal and following the other principles of the Hunger Free Forever program will also help to ensure that your resting metabolism is preserved even if you lose significant amounts of weight.

CALCULATING YOUR DAILY CALORIC NEEDS

Although we use sophisticated equipment to measure basal metabolic rate, most dieticians and healthcare providers use a simple equation known as the Harris-Benedict Equation to estimate resting calorie expenditure. You can use these equations to estimate your basal metabolic rate:

For men: $(13.75 \times$ weight in kg$) + (5 \times$ height in cm$) - (6.76 \times$ age in yrs$) + 66$

For women: $(9.56 \times$ weight in kg$) + (1.85 \times$ height in cm$) - (4.68 \times$ age in yrs$) + 655$

1 pound = 0.45 kilogram (kg)

1 inch = 2.54 centimeters (cm)

Once you have calculated your basal metabolic rate, your daily caloric requirements to maintain your body weight can be estimated below:

(continued on next page)

Activity level	Multiply basal metabolism by this amount to estimate total calories required
Bed rest	1.2
Sedentary	1.3
Active	1.4
Very active	1.5

Here is an example for a forty-year-old, 5'6" woman weighing 170 pounds:

$(9.56 \times 76.5) + (1.85 \times 167.54) - (4.68 \times 40) + 655 = 1{,}509$ calories.

If she was sedentary, her BMR would be $(1{,}509 \times 1.3) = 1{,}962$ calories.

If she was very active, her BMR would be $(1{,}509 \times 1.5) = 2{,}264$ calories.

THE THYROID: THE MASTER GLAND OF METABOLISM

Before we go too much further in discussing metabolism, it is important for you and your doctor to make sure that your thyroid gland is functioning properly. This small gland is just about the same size and shape and is in the same location as a small bow tie. The thyroid gland secretes two hormones that are crucial for regulating metabolism: triiodothyronine (T_3) and thyroxine (T_4). The numbers refer to the number of iodine atoms each molecule of hormone contains. T_3 is more potent than T_4, but most of the thyroid hormone in the body is in the form of T_4.

Low levels of thyroid hormone, or hypothyroidism, is a very common problem affecting perhaps one out of ten women and a smaller percentage of men. If your thyroid activity is reduced, your metabolism is significantly impaired and you will have a very difficult time losing weight. Hence, it is important to make sure your thyroid is working properly. However, we should point out that taking excess thyroid hormone does not promote weight loss and is linked to loss of muscle mass and bone. The key is to make sure that you are secreting enough thyroid hormone, but not too much.

Since thyroid hormones affect every cell of the body, a deficiency will usually result in a large number of signs and symptoms including low body temperature, intolerance to cold, weight gain or an inability to lose weight, depression, lack of concentration, hair loss, and fatigue. If you have any of these symptoms, it is important to check with your doctor to rule out an underactive thyroid.

Your doctor can conduct a blood test that measures thyroid hormone levels. The test assesses the quantity of T_4 and T_3 hormones and determines how well the body's cells respond to the hormones by measuring the level of thyroid stimulating hormone (TSH), a chemical released by the pituitary gland. High levels of TSH indicate that the cells of the body are not receiving adequate thyroid hormone. As a result, the pituitary goes into overdrive, frantically trying to signal the thyroid to step up its hormone output.

The medical treatment of hypothyroidism, in all but its most mild forms, involves the use of thyroid hormone, which may be in the form of desiccated thyroid or synthetic thyroid hormone, such as Synthroid or levothyroxine. It may take a month or two to stabilize the dosage. After that, periodic evaluations are based on the individual patient's needs and are recommended to be carried out at least once a year.

COMMON SIGNS AND SYMPTOMS OF HYPOTHYROIDISM:

- Depression
- Difficulty in losing weight
- Dry skin
- Headaches
- Lethargy or fatigue
- Heavy or irregular periods
- Recurrent infections
- Sensitivity to cold

THE MISSING LINK IN ENERGY CONSUMPTION

Although the resting metabolism of overweight or obese people is generally somewhat higher than those with normal weight, the amount of energy consumed through activity can vary tremendously. Activity energy expenditure refers to the energy consumed through planned exercise as well as the energy consumed in every other activity during your day. We discussed the importance of exercise in the last chapter. However, breakthrough research at the Mayo Clinic has uncovered an important missing link in the understanding of metabolism in overweight and obese people. Under the direction of James Levine, M.D., the Mayo Clinic has conducted the most extensive investigation of non-exercise energy expenditure, also referred to as non-exercise activity thermogenesis or NEAT.

It is common sense that some people burn more calories than others in their occupation or activities of daily living. However, the Mayo Clinic researchers have discovered that there is a fundamental difference between normal-weight and obese subjects in terms of how much energy they expend through NEAT in a given day. Dr. Levine and his colleagues have shown that lean and obese individuals are different in the energy dedicated to the maintenance of posture, activities of daily living, and even fidgeting. As mentioned in the previous chapter, a person of normal weight typically sits 150 fewer minutes each day, and burns 350 more calories per day from the collective impact of numerous small activities and movements than someone who is overweight. Burning 350 calories per day is equivalent to about 40 pounds of fat in one year, so this is a very important factor in long-term weight control. Although this difference may be genetically preprogrammed to some extent, it can certainly be modified with some effort.

A NEAT Way to Lose Weight

Mayo Clinic researchers point out that long-term weight control may be easier to maintain by focusing more on increasing NEAT than by planned exercise. Certainly both are important, but the potential of NEAT is quite extraordinary. For instance, Dr. Levine's lab has set up a model office where workers each stand on a treadmill with a special computer stand that allows them to type, talk on the phone, and conduct their daily work while they walk at 0.7 miles per hour. People report that it is easy to get used to this very slow pace and they actually experience less fatigue, increased mental clarity, and better work performance. Walking in this way burns an extra 100 to 150 calories per hour, or up to 1,000 calories per day. This is as many calories as an elite athlete might burn during a training session for an Olympic event.

Increase Your NEAT and Burn Calories

Although the idea of treadmill desks or recumbent bikes built into computer workstations may be in our future, there are many things we can do to increase the calories we expend through NEAT. Increasing the amount of unstructured activity in your daily routine can potentially help you achieve a healthful weight as effectively as working out at the gym. The following are a few suggestions to get you started:

Get out of your chair.

Standing and doing nothing burns about two calories per minute, compared with one calorie for sitting and doing nothing. Stretch frequently while you stand to increase the calorie expenditure even further.

Change your work environment.

Although a treadmill with attached computer may not be practical, an adjustable-height worktable that allows you to stand and work is easy to find and provides a surprisingly comfortable way to work for at least part of your day.

Add activity wherever you can.

Walk whenever you can. Take the stairs instead of the elevator. Lift things, do the dishes, work in the yard. Remember, every little bit of activity adds to your daily calorie burn.

Pace while handling phone calls.

Use a headset and pace when you talk on the phone. One minute of pacing burns three or more calories. Remember, every calorie burned is one less stored.

In general, sit rather than lie down, stand rather than sit, pace rather than stand, walk rather than pace.

Even though the calories burned per hour from these kinds of activities seems small, over days, months, and years they can amount to hundred of thousands of calories and many pounds of fat.

Food Burns Calories, Too!

Apart from resting metabolism and activity energy expenditure, the body also burns calories every time you eat. This is referred to as the thermic effects of food or the thermogenic effects of food. In order for you to use the calories from your food, digestion and processing of nutrients has a certain cost in the form of calories. As well, it is vital that your body maintain itself in a narrow temperature range so it has to spend a certain amount of calories on producing heat.

The thermic effect of food can vary quite substantially. Protein is actually the hardest food for your body to process and utilize. Therefore, your body wastes 20 to 30 percent of the calories in protein in its processing and the release of heat. This is one of the best reasons to eat sufficient protein with each meal. On the other hand, carbohydrates are utilized more efficiently by the body so that 5 to 10 percent of the calories in carbohydrates are wasted in processing and heat. Fat is the most efficient source of energy for your body, because only zero to 3 percent of the calories in fat are used in processing and heat. This is why fat in excess tends to go right onto your waistline.

Spread Your Calories Throughout the Day

One of the most important things you can do to ensure that your body burns a significant number of calories as heat is to spread your calories throughout the day. Skipping meals lowers your resting metabolism and makes it more likely that your body will store the extra calories eaten later as fat. A low-glycemic impact, high-protein breakfast is the most important food of the day. When you skip breakfast, you are telling your body that you are starving today and your metabolic rate will likely be lower for the rest of the day. When you start the day with a hearty breakfast, you are telling your body that there is plenty of food, so it tends to expend more of the calories you eat that day as heat. It is also important to follow breakfast with healthy snacks, lunches, and a relatively light evening meal.

Diet-Induced Thermogenesis in Lean Versus Obese Individuals

In lean individuals, a meal may stimulate up to a 40 percent increase in heat production. In contrast, the very same meal consumed by an overweight or obese individual will likely produce only a 10 percent or less increase in heat production. In the overweight or obese individual, the food energy is stored instead of being converted to heat.

Consistent with other aspects of the tendency toward obesity, the major factor for the decreased thermogenesis in overweight and obese people is insulin insensitivity. Once again, enhancing insulin sensitivity becomes extremely important. In this case, improving the action of insulin goes a long way in reestablishing normal thermogenesis in overweight and obese individuals. Furthermore, there is a track of preliminary research showing that the reduction in diet-induced thermogenesis due to insulin resistance leads to impairment of satiety, which in turn leads to increased food intake. In other words, adequate diet-induced thermogenesis appears to be critical in turning off the "feed me" switch in the brain. Therefore, measures that increase diet-induced thermogenesis are also likely to lead to greater satiety.

In addition to insulin insensitivity, there are other key factors that determine the level of diet-induced thermogenesis. For example, the amount of brown fat an individual carries has a major impact. Most fat in the body is white fat consisting of an energy reserve containing fats (triglycerides) housed in one large droplet. Tissue composed of white fat will look white or pale yellow. In contrast, brown fat cells are special fat cells that contain multiple compartments instead of the one big compartment of the white fat cell. The triglycerides are localized in smaller droplets surrounding numerous energy producing compartments known as mitochondria. An extensive blood vessel network along with the density of the mitochondria gives the tissue its brown appearance, as well as its impressive capacity to burn fat. In other tissues of the body, including white fat, the loss of chemical energy as heat is minimized. In contrast, brown fat wastes energy by burning higher amounts of fat and giving off more heat. As such, brown fat plays a major role in diet-induced thermogenesis.

Some theories suggest that lean people have a higher percentage of brown fat to white fat than overweight and obese individuals. There is evidence to support this theory. The amount of brown fat in modern humans is extremely small (estimates are 0.5 to 5 percent of total body weight), but because of its profound effect on diet-induced thermogenesis, as little as one ounce of brown fat (0.1 percent of body weight) could make the difference between maintaining body weight and putting on an extra 10 pounds per year.

Lean individuals also tend to respond differently to excess calories than overweight and obese individuals. In one experiment, lean individuals were fattened up. In order for these subjects to maintain the excess weight, they had to increase their caloric intake by 50 percent over their previous intake. The opposite appears to be the case in overweight and formerly overweight and obese individuals. In addition to requiring fewer calories to maintain their weight, studies have shown that in order to maintain their reduced weight, they needed to restrict their caloric intake to approximately 25 percent less than a lean person of similar weight and body size.

The Effect of Dietary Fat on Thermogenesis

Individuals predisposed to obesity because of decreased diet-induced thermogenesis have been shown to be extremely sensitive to marked weight gain when consuming a high-fat diet, compared to lean individuals. However, individuals predisposed are not only more sensitive to the weight-gain promoting effects of a high-fat diet, they tend to consume much more dietary fat than lean individuals, and they tend to exercise less. Let's take a look at this equation:

Predisposition to obesity due to decreased diet-induced thermogenesis
+ Increased sensitivity to weight-gain promoting effects of a high-fat diet

+ Consumption of a high-fat diet
+ Lack of exercise
= Obesity

Perhaps more important than consuming a low-fat diet to promote weight loss is making sure that the diet is composed of the right types of fats. Specifically, monounsaturated fats and sources of medium chain triglycerides can help promote diet-induced thermogenesis and weight loss. We have highlighted the importance of monounsaturated fats in improving insulin sensitivity and promoting satiety. In addition to these mechanisms, the monounsaturated fats in nuts, seeds, and olive oil have been shown to produce an increase in diet-induced thermogenesis.

The best source of medium chain triglycerides is coconut oil. Coconuts, like most nuts, contain significant amounts of fat, but unlike other nuts, which contain mostly monounsaturated fat, the fat provided by coconuts is almost all in the form of health-promoting medium chain triglycerides (MCTs). The MCTs in coconut oil are saturated fats that range in length from 6 to 12 carbon chains. In contrast, the long chain triglycerides (LCTs) found in most other foods are 18 to 24 carbons long. The LCTs are not only the most abundant fats found in nature, they are also the form of storage fat in our bodies as well. This difference in length determines how MCTs and LCTs are utilized. Unlike regular fats, MCTs consumed in moderate amounts do not appear to cause weight gain. In fact, they promote weight loss.

Here is a good analogy: LCTs are like heavy, wet logs that you put on a small campfire. Keep adding the logs, and soon you have more logs than fire. MCTs, by comparison, are like rolled up newspaper soaked in gasoline. They not only burn brightly, they burn up the wet logs as well. In one study, the thermogenic effect of a high-calorie diet containing 40 percent fat as MCTs was compared to one containing the same level of LCTs. The thermic effect (calories wasted six hours after a meal) of the MCTs was almost twice as high as the LCTs. With MCTs, 120 calories were used, compared to 66 calories from LCTs over the six hours. A follow-up study demonstrated that MCT oil given over a six-day period can increase diet-induced thermogenesis by 50 percent.

In another study, researchers compared the effects of single meals of 400 calories composed entirely of MCTs or LCTs. The thermogenic effect of MCTs over six hours was 300 percent higher than the LCTs meal. Since the MCTs went directly to the liver and were burned, they had no effect on the blood fat level. However, the LCTs elevated blood fats by 68 percent. Researchers concluded that "long-term substitution of medium chain triglycerides for long chain triglycerides [MCT for LCT] would produce weight loss if energy intake remained constant." So if you simply substitute coconut oil for sources of LCTs in your diet, you are going to lose weight. We recommend substituting coconut oil for butter and other oils to be used in salad dressings, spreads, and for low-temperature cooking.

Thermogenic Formulas

Herbal formulas containing mixtures of caffeine and ephedrine were once the most popular weight-loss products in the nutritional supplement industry. There was no question that these products worked to promote diet-induced thermogenesis and weight loss, but they were abused by some and side effects were common. When ephedrine was linked to several deaths due mainly to abuse, it ultimately led to the banning of ephedrine-containing supplements by the FDA.

Ephedrine has been replaced in many thermogenic formulas by synephrine, a compound from bitter orange (*Citrus aurantium*) that possesses similar thermogenic effects to ephedrine. In the body, synephrine is able to bind to the same types of receptor sites on fat cells as ephedrine. The beta-3 receptor is the most important one for weight management. When either ephedrine or synephrine binds to the beta-3 receptor, it causes fat cells to burn more calories as heat (thermogenesis) by breaking down fat (lipolysis). The advantage of synephrine is that it does not stimulate the other receptor sites (alpha-1, beta-1, and beta-2 receptors) to the same degree as ephedrine. Yet, there is growing concern regarding the safety of synephrine. Until safety issues are clarified, we do not recommend that you use synephrine.

The Thermogenic Effect of Green Tea Catechins

Green tea has shown considerable effects as a thermogenic aid. In addition to its caffeine content, the catechins or polyphenols in green tea also exert a thermogenic effect. Both green tea and black tea are derived from the same plant, *Camellia sinensis*. The difference between green and black teas results from the manufacturing process. Green tea is produced by lightly steaming the fresh-cut leaf. Steaming prevents enzymes in the tea leaves from converting the beneficial polyphenols. To produce black tea, the leaves are simply dried and the beneficial polyphenols are allowed to oxidize and form larger complexes, known as tannins.

Green tea is one of the most important health promoting beverages you can drink. Regular green tea consumption is linked to a reduced risk for heart attacks and strokes as well as most forms of cancer, particularly breast and prostate cancer. The health benefits of green tea are due to the presence of molecules known as polyphenols or catechins, the most active of which is epigallocatechin gallate (EGCg). While green tea can be consumed as a beverage, to get the weight-loss promoting benefits you will need to use green tea extracts concentrated for EGCg and other catechins at an effective dosage. A regular cup of green tea may contain anywhere from 30 to 80mg of catechins (as well as 30 to 50mg of caffeine). Green tea extracts are now commercially available that contain 70 to 99 percent catechin content without the caffeine. In order to produce real effect in weight loss, the intake of catechins must be in excess of 540mg daily.

COCA-COLA LAUNCHES GREEN TEA BEVERAGE

In November 2006, Coca-Cola's Enviga green tea beverage hit the shelves. Enviga is a joint venture between Coke and Nestlé. It is marketed as "The Calorie Burner" with the additional claim that it will burn an extra 60 to 100 calories per day. Are these claims true? Perhaps, but you have to look a little deeper to see at what price this effect comes.

Coke points to a single study of Enviga, undertaken in the University of Lausanne in collaboration with the Nestlé Research Center in Lausanne, Switzerland. The study showed that consuming the

(continued on next page)

equivalent of three Enviga beverages over the course of the day increased the burn of calories by 106 calories. Enviga does contain 90mg of EGCg and 100mg of caffeine per 12-ounce can. So drinking three cans per day will provide 270mg of EGCg and 300mg of caffeine (about the same amount as in two cups of coffee). The study tested thirty-one people aged between 18 and 35. All of the test subjects were in the normal weight range, so it is not known what effect Enviga may have in overweight and obese individuals.

Hypothetically, let's say these results are accurate. In order to burn one pound of fat (3,500 calories), you would need to drink 105 cans of Enviga for 35 days straight. Not only is that expensive (about $150 over the 35 days), but Enviga contains artificial sweeteners and other ingredients that are probably not wise to consume in such large quantities. Hence, if you are looking for the weight-loss promoting effects of green tea catechins and EGCg, it may be more effective, healthier, and less costly to look at other options, such as green tea extracts.

So how much weight can you expect to lose by taking green tea catechins? In one of the best designed studies, eighty subjects were given a drink providing either 126mg of catechins or 588mg of catechins for twelve weeks. The group getting the lower dosage of catechins did not experience any significant weight loss, but in the higher dosage group there was an average weight loss of about four pounds, a little more than a pound a week. The decrease in body weight was almost entirely due to loss of body fat and the loss of body fat was almost exclusively due to a loss in visceral (abdominal) fat.

Several mechanisms are thought to be responsible for the weight-loss producing effects of green tea catechins. Not only do these compounds promote diet-induced thermogenesis; they have also been shown to reduce the formation of fat cells, increase the burning of fat for energy (not just heat), decrease fat absorption, and increase the levels of fat cell–derived hormones such as leptin and adiponectin that enhance the action of insulin. As such, we advocate incorporating green tea beverages and supplements into your daily routine. Remember, to see much benefit in weight loss, you need to ingest about 600mg of catechins each day.

To Burn Fat and Support Liver Health

The liver is the second-largest organ in the body and is the largest gland. It is critically involved in all aspects of metabolism and plays a central role in fat, protein, and carbohydrate processing. When liver function is impaired, the ability to burn fat properly and thermogenesis are also impaired. Many overweight individuals develop what is known as a fatty liver or nonalcoholic steatohepatitis (NASH), and as a result show signs of a sluggish liver resulting in a sluggish metabolism.

As you lose weight, it is very important to support liver function. The best way to support the liver is to avoid putting undue stress on it while simultaneously providing the key nutritional building blocks that it needs to function properly. Some simple guidelines: don't smoke; drink little or no alcohol; avoid drugs that can harm the liver (even acetaminophen or Tylenol); and do your best to avoid harmful chemicals, especially cleaning solvents and pesticides. The most important dietary guidelines for supporting good liver function are also those that support good general health: avoid saturated fats, refined sugar, and alcohol; drink at least forty-eight ounces of water each day; and consume plenty of vegetables and legumes for their high fiber and nutrient content.

Certain foods are particularly helpful in supporting liver health because they contain the nutrients your body needs to produce and activate the dozens of enzymes within the liver involved in the various phases of detoxification of harmful chemicals. Such foods include:

- Garlic, legumes, onions, eggs, and other foods with a high sulfur content
- Good sources of water-soluble fibers, such as pears, oat bran, apples, and legumes
- Cabbage-family vegetables, especially broccoli, Brussels sprouts, and cabbage

- Artichokes, beets, carrots, dandelion greens, and many herbs and spices such as turmeric, cinnamon, red pepper, ginger, and licorice
- Green foods like wheat grass juice, dehydrated barley grass juice, chlorella, and spirulina.

CHAPTER SUMMARY

- Metabolism plays a central role in weight loss and even a more vital role in the long-term maintenance of healthy weight.
- Metabolism refers to the breakdown of food into energy that is used to sustain life.
- Studies have shown that rather than having low metabolism, overweight and obese people often underestimate the amount of food they eat by as much as 30 percent.
- It is important to rule out low thyroid function to succeed in weight loss and sustain overall good health.
- A conscious effort to increase non-exercise energy activity thermogenesis (NEAT) may turn out to be a better strategy than exercise for many people trying to lose weight.
- Diet-induced thermogenesis is the method in which the body "wastes" calories.
- The major factor for the decreased thermogenesis in overweight and obese people is insulin insensitivity.
- Brown fat cells burn fat.
- Lean people have a higher percentage of brown fat to white fat than overweight and obese individuals.
- Studies have shown that in order to maintain their reduced weight, formerly obese persons must restrict their caloric intake to approximately 25 percent less than a lean person of similar weight and body size.
- Monounsaturated fats and sources of medium chain triglycerides can help promote diet-induced thermogenesis and weight loss.
- The health benefits of green tea are due to the presence of molecules known as polyphenols or catechins, the most active of which is epigallocatechin gallate (EGCg).

- Green tea catechins at a dosage of 588mg per day produced an average weight loss of four pounds in one twelve-week study.
- Green tea extract has been shown to reduce the formation of fat cells, increase the burning of fat for energy (not just heat), decrease fat absorption, and increase the levels of leptin and adiponectin.
- Supporting healthy liver function is critical in burning fat.
- Adding red pepper as well as garlic and ginger to your diet is a safe, natural way to support the liver.

9

PROGRAM YOURSELF

FOR SUCCESS

Rather than using psychological therapies in an attempt to reduce food intake, our focus is to utilize techniques that promote a positive self-image and high self-esteem. Let's face it, there is tremendous stigma attached to being overweight or obese that causes a lot of psychological trauma. Fashion trends, insurance programs, college placements, and job opportunities all discriminate against the obese or overweight person. Consequently, the obese or overweight person learns many self-defeating and self-degrading attitudes. They are led to believe that fat is "bad," which often results in a vicious cycle of low self-esteem, depression, overeating for consolation, increased weight gain, social rejection, and further lowering of self-esteem.

Achieving permanent weight loss with the Hunger Free Forever program has a phenomenal effect on increasing self-esteem and promoting a healthy positive mental attitude. In fact, this positive effect is supported by research. A detailed analysis of 117 weight-loss studies has confirmed that successful weight loss is associated with significant improvement in self-esteem. Interestingly, test subjects also showed improvement in mood with lowered scores for depression independent of weight loss. In other words, just being included in the clinical study was enough to improve mood and depression.

Rather than waiting to have healthy self-esteem until you actually lose weight, you can take steps to build self-esteem and program yourself for the success right now. The following success exercise program is just as essential to your weight-loss plan as physical exercise. To get started, you will need to get a notebook that will become your personal journal. A journal is a powerful tool to help you stay in touch with your feelings, thoughts, and emotions. You can construct your own journal or visit www.hungerfreeforever.com, go to the Downloads page, and click on Success Journal. In chapter 10, we provide the instructions for keeping your journal.

The following exercises are designed to help you learn how to adopt healthier attitudes. They will provide the foundation for building your increased self-esteem, and your personal journal will serve as a testimony to your success.

EXERCISE #1: CREATING A POSITIVE GOAL STATEMENT

Learning to set goals in a way that results in a positive experience is critical to your success. The following guidelines can be used to set any goal, whether short or long term, including your desired weight. You can use goal setting to create a success cycle—a succession of positive achievements. Achieving goals helps you feel better about yourself and the better you feel about yourself, the more likely you are to achieve your goals. Success breeds success.

1. State the goal in positive terms; do not use any negative words in your goal statement. For example it is better to say "I enjoy eating healthy, low-calorie, nutritious foods," than "I will not eat sugar, candy, ice cream, and other fattening foods."
2. Make your short-term goals attainable and realistic. Again, short-term goals can be used to create a success cycle and positive self-image. Little successes add up to make a major difference in the way you feel about yourself.
3. Be specific. The clearer your goal is defined, the more likely you are to reach it. What is the exact weight you desire? What are the body fat percentage or measurements you desire? Clearly define what it is you want to achieve.
4. State the goal in present tense, not future tense. In order to

reach your goal, you have to believe you have already attained it. As noted psychologist Dr. Wayne Dyer says "You'll see it, when you believe it." You must literally program yourself to achieve the goal. See and feel yourself having already achieved the goal and success will be yours. Remember always state your goal in the present tense.

Short- and Long-Term Goal Statements

Use the guidelines above to construct both a short- and long-term positive goal statement.

For example, a short-term goal statement could be: "My body is strong and beautiful. I feel good about myself and my body. I am losing 2 pounds a week and I feel fantastic!" And a long-term goal statement could be: "I am a size 6. I feel beautiful, thin, and full of energy."

Any voyage begins with one step and is followed by many other steps. Short-term goals can be used to help you achieve those long-term results described in your positive goal statement. Get in the habit of asking yourself the following question each morning and evening: What must I do today to achieve my long-term goal?

EXERCISE #2: ASK POSITIVE QUESTIONS

According to Anthony Robbins, author of the bestselling books *Unlimited Power* and *Awaken the Giant Within*, the quality of your life is equal to the quality of the questions you habitually ask yourself. This belief is based on the assumption that whatever question you ask your brain, it will answer. If you want to have a better life, you need to ask better questions. To help you achieve not only your desired weight, but also a happier life, get in the habit of asking yourself the following questions on a consistent basis.

The Morning Questions

1. What am I most happy about in my life right now? Why does that make me happy? How does that make me feel?
2. What am I most excited about in my life right now? Why does that make me excited? How does that make me feel?

3. What am I most grateful about in my life right now? Why does that make me grateful? How does that make me feel?
4. What am I enjoying most in my life right now? What about that do I enjoy? How does that make me feel?
5. What am I committed to in my life right now? Why am I committed to that? How does that make me feel?
6. What must I do today to achieve my long-term goal?

The Evening Questions
1. What have I given today? In what ways have I been a giver today?
2. What did I learn today?
3. In what ways was today a perfect day?
4. Repeat morning questions.

The Problem or Challenge Questions
1. What is right or great about this problem?
2. What is not perfect yet?
3. What am I willing to do to make it the way I want?
4. How can I enjoy doing the things necessary to make it the way I want?

EXERCISE #3: POSITIVE AFFIRMATIONS

An affirmation is a statement of fact that can make an imprint on the subconscious mind to create a healthy, positive self-image. In addition, affirmations can actually fuel the changes you desire. Here are some guidelines for creating your own affirmations:

1. Always phrase an affirmation in the present tense.
2. Always phrase the affirmation in a positive way and stay tuned to the positive feelings that are generated.
3. Keep the affirmation short and simple, but full of feeling.
4. Be creative.
5. Imagine yourself really experiencing what you are affirming.
6. Make the affirmation personal and full of meaning.

Here are some examples of positive affirmations:

- I am a whole and complete person.
- I am in control of my life.
- I am an open channel of love and joy.
- I am filled with peace and wisdom.
- I am good to my body.
- I am growing stronger every day.
- I am healthier and thinner.

Using the above guidelines and examples, write down five affirmations regarding eating healthful meals and five affirmations about physical activity. State these affirmations aloud for a total of five minutes each day. Choose a location that is comfortable and quiet, and a time when you will not be interrupted or disturbed. Sit or lie in a comfortable position. Begin by taking ten deep breaths, inhaling to a count of one, holding for a count of two, and exhaling to a count of four.

CHAPTER SUMMARY

- Achieving permanent weight loss leads to an increase in self-esteem and positive attitude.
- Rather than waiting to have healthy self-esteem until you actually lose weight, you can take immediate steps to build self-esteem and program yourself for the success.
- Learning to set goals in a way that results in a positive experience is critical to your success.
- The quality of your life is equal to the quality of the questions you habitually ask yourself.
- Positive affirmations can fuel the changes you desire.

10

How to Live the Hunger Free Forever Program

Long-term weight-loss success is based upon achieving five key goals:

- Effectively decrease appetite, leading to a reduction of calories consumed
- Normalize and stabilize blood glucose levels
- Increase metabolism and the burning of fat, while preserving lean muscle mass
- Reset the mechanisms that control individual fat cell size and body weight
- Make food and lifestyle choices that promote ideal body weight and create a healthier relationship with food

The Hunger Free Forever program effectively weaves each of these five key goals into an easy-to-follow daily program. By following the guidelines outlined in this chapter, you can look forward to a lifetime of appetite and weight control.

CREATE A SUCCESS JOURNAL

We recommend creating a journal to provide a detailed account of your feelings, thoughts, and emotions as you embark on the Hunger Free Forever program. You can construct your own journal or you can go to www.hungerfreeforever.com and go to the Downloads page and click on Success Journal. Here are the instructions for keeping your journal.

Each morning fill in the date, write out your goal statement, and sign your commitment to this goal. Next, make a checklist to include the following so that you perform all of these essential items every day:

- ☐ Write out goal statement
- ☐ Ask morning questions
- ☐ Recite positive affirmations
- ☐ Breakfast
- ☐ Midmorning snack
- ☐ Lunch
- ☐ Midafternoon snack
- ☐ Dinner
- ☐ Evening snack
- ☐ Physical exercise
- ☐ Relaxation exercise

In order to help you to achieve your goal, we suggest you also document every food item you eat and everything you drink, including snacks. Doing so helps you gain better control of your intake. It will also help to minimize cheating. Several studies have shown that keeping a food diary greatly improves your chance of success at weight loss.

Lastly, at the end of the day we want you to give yourself a grade:

A+ I ate all the right foods and didn't cheat or overeat today.
B Mostly kept to my eating goals. I'm still losing weight.
C Cheated a bit or overate, but not too badly. I probably didn't gain or lose weight.
D Cheated or overate and probably gained some weight.
F Fell off track and likely gained weight today.

Obviously, we want you to be an A+ student and our plan sets you up to be one. You will notice that we have included a total of six meals.

In addition to breakfast, lunch, and dinner, we want you to enjoy three low-calorie, nutritious snacks. Why? To lose weight, you absolutely must make your body and brain feel like they are well nourished. If you get hungry, you are more likely to overeat. We want you to feel satisfied at all times.

In addition to the daily diary, we want you to fill out a weekly progress report. You can download this form from www.hungerfree forever.com. If you want to make your own progress report, simply record your weight at the same time each day. At the end of the week, add up all recorded weights and divide by seven to give you your average weight. Subtract that number from your starting weight. Next, subtract your weight loss this week from the average weight from the previous week to determine this week's weight loss.

It is also a good idea to measure your waist and hips each week and note the changes there as well. Determine the waist-to-hip ratio by dividing the waist measurement by the hip measurement. For men, a ratio of .90 or less is considered desirable. For women, a ratio of .80 or less is considered desirable. To measure waist circumference comfortably, measure the distance around the area one inch above the belly button. To measure hip circumference, comfortably measure the distance around the largest protrusion of the buttocks.

PGX–AN ABSOLUTE MUST FOR EFFECTIVE AND PERMANENT WEIGHT LOSS

In our clinical experience, we have discovered a very important fact: The key ingredient to successful weight loss is the ingestion of 2.5 to 5 grams of PGX at major meals and perhaps at least twice more for those with an appetite more difficult to tame. Initially, we spent a lot of time in the clinic educating our patients on the importance of diet and menu planning, but then we found out that we actually got better results with our patients when we simply stressed using PGX along with becoming more conscious of what and how much you are eating. That said, we provide the full program in this chapter just as we have utilized it in our clinical experience. However, don't lose sight of the fact that the key to real success is using PGX liberally.

PGX is available in capsules (either hard or soft gelatin), as a zero-calorie drink mix, as granules to be added into food and beverages, and in a sophisticated low-carbohydrate, very low-glycemic index meal replacement drink containing undenatured whey protein, natural flavors, and sweeteners along with vitamins and minerals. The primary supplier of PGX is Natural Factors, who offers PGX in their SlimStyles family of products for weight loss. These products can be found in health food stores throughout North America or via a number of e-tailers on the Internet. To find a store near you, please go to www.slimstyles.com. For more information about the science behind PGX and how to use it most effectively, see appendix D or go to www.PGX.com. Here is a quick checklist of how to use PGX in your daily diet:

- Take SlimStyles Weight Loss Drink Mix with PGX at least once per day as a meal replacement. (Note: this product is called SlimStyles Weight Loss Meal Replacement Drink Mix with PGX in Canada.)
- Before meals when you are not using SlimStyles Weight Loss Drink Mix with PGX as a meal replacement, you must take PGX. If using PGX granules, take 2.5 to 5 grams in a glass of water. Note, SlimStyx from Natural Factors provides 2.5 grams of PGX in a convenient small tube-shaped packet that is excellent to bring along with you when you are eating out. If you are using the PGX in soft gelatin capsules, less PGX is required in this form. Take three to six soft gelatin capsules with a glass of water before meals.
- Use PGX granules or soft gel capsules when hungry between meals.
- Follow the menu suggestions.
- Drink water! While it is wise to drink at least 48 ounces of water daily, it is vital to do so when taking PGX.

DAILY PLAN

Following is a template daily food plan, from which all of your menu plans can be built:

Breakfast Two scoops of SlimStyles Weight Loss Drink Mix blended with 12 to 16 ounces of water for a low-glycemic, high-volumetric

How to Use SlimStyles Products

SlimStyles Weight Loss Drink Mix (2 scoops = 5 grams of PGX plus other nutrients)

- For a calorie-restricted diet and to achieve your weight-loss needs, have the SlimStyles Weight Loss Drink Mix at breakfast and lunch, followed by a healthy balanced dinner.
- Breakfast is the most important meal of the day, so the meal replacement is great for those who don't like eating a full meal for breakfast.
- Each serving provides only 220 calories.
- Contains high-quality whey protein, medium chain triglycerides, and important micronutrients for health.
- Because this is a meal replacement, it has all the nutrients you need for a full meal in a flash. Because you don't have to buy food for the meal that is replaced, this can be a very economical way to get a very nutritious meal.

SlimStyles PGX Granules (1 scoop = 5 grams of PGX)

- PGX unflavored granules can be added directly to moist food and beverages.
- PGX granules are calorie free.
- Add PGX granules to your meals or with snacks when you know your appetite is strong.
- Don't forget to drink 8 to 12 ounces of water with each serving.
- Many of our patients mix PGX granules in water or juice—V8 juice is a very popular, low-calorie choice—and take this right before their meal to increase their sense of fullness with less food.

SlimStyles SlimStyx PGX Granules (1 packet = 2.5 grams of PGX)

- These packets are convenient to carry with you so that you can easily add PGX to water or other beverages and food when you are on the go.

(continued on next page)

- They are perfect for adding to a bottle of water.
- Take one or two SlimStyx with each meal. Some of our patients find it very effective to take one SlimStyx in water or juice right before their meal and one more SlimStyx right after their meal.

SlimStyles PGX Soft Gelatin Capsules (2 capsules = 1.5 grams of PGX)

- This product provides pure PGX emulsified with medium chain triglycerides (MCTs).
- Provides enhanced viscosity compared to other PGX products because of the MCTs.
- Lower dosages of PGX are required when using this form.
- When strapped for time, traveling, or out for dinner, these soft gel capsules are the most convenient way to take PGX.
- Take three to six capsules fifteen to twenty minutes before meals.

SlimStyles PGX Hard Gelatin Capsules
(5 capsules = 2.5 grams of PGX)

- Since so many capsules need to be consumed, we recommend other PGX products before this one.
- We suggest taking up to five capsules before you eat and up to five capsules after. Some people find that a total of only five capsules with each meal reduces their appetite quite successfully.
- When strapped for time, traveling, or out for dinner, the capsules can be an easy way to take PGX, but we recommend the soft gel version.

SlimStyles PGX Appetite Control Fiber Blend
(2 scoops = 5 grams of PGX)

- An orange-flavored blend of PGX granules. It provides taste with no extra calories when taking PGX granules in water.

breakfast. A small amount (e.g., ½ cup) of frozen fruit can be added and mixed in the blender, if desired.

Snack A 100- to 150-calorie snack focusing on low-glycemic, high-volumetric foods.

Before Lunch 2.5 to 5 grams of PGX granules in a glass of water or V8-type juice.

Lunch A low-glycemic, high-volumetric lunch or simply have another SlimStyles Weight Loss Drink Mix drink

Snack A 100- to 150-calorie snack focusing on low-glycemic, high-volumetric foods.

Before Dinner 2.5 to 5 grams of PGX granules in a glass of water 5 to 15 minutes before dinner.

Dinner A low-glycemic, high-volumetric meal. For instance: One serving (50 to 100 grams) of baked chicken breast, salmon, lean meat, or tofu; a medium salad with olive oil and natural herbs and spices; one serving (1 to 2 cups) of a cooked nonstarchy vegetable; and ½ cup berries for dessert. **NOTE:** As an alternative for dessert, make up ½ serving of SlimStyles Weight Loss Drink Mix before dinner and place in fridge. In forty to sixty minutes, it turns into a delicious and appetite suppressing pudding!

Evening Snack or Tea A 100- to 150-calorie snack focusing on low-glycemic, high-volumetric foods or, better yet, one or two cups of herbal tea (no caffeine).

A FEW STAPLE FOODS FOR HEALTHY WEIGHT LOSS
- Oatmeal
- Yams (and sweet potatoes)
- Brown rice
- Green, yellow, orange, purple, or red fibrous, nutrient dense vegetables
- Fresh fruit (tropical fruits in moderation)
- Nonfat dairy products
- High-quality whey protein
- Legumes (beans)
- Chicken and turkey breast, skinless and boneless, including ground chicken or turkey, but choose the leanest varieties available
- Eggs (including egg substitutes like Egg Beaters) and egg whites, fish, and very lean red meats

Breakfast

The best breakfast that we can recommend for effective weight loss or management is the SlimStyles Weight Loss Drink Mix. We designed this product to promote satiety and increase metabolism. Two scoops provide 5 grams of PGX, 19 grams of whey protein, 2.3 grams of medium chain triglycerides, and more than thirty other nutrients, vitamins, and minerals to support healthy metabolism. And it tastes great.

The most important reasons why this drink mix provides the perfect way to start the day are that it is extremely filling and it exerts a tremendous blood sugar stabilizing effect. We have done our own intensive research on the SlimStyles Weight Loss Drink with our patients. To verify our results because they were so phenomenal, we had Sydney University's Glycemic Index Research Service (SUGIRS) perform an evaluation. As you can see below, the drink mix produces an incredible effect on stabilizing blood sugar levels for at least two hours.

This graph demonstrates that the SlimStyles Weight Loss Drink Mix does not raise blood sugar levels above fasting levels. So if your fasting blood sugar level was 90mg/dl upon arising and you had a serv-

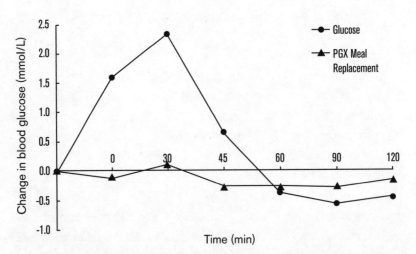

Figure 10.1.–Effect of SlimStyles Weight Loss Drink Mix on Blood Sugar Levels as Evaluated by Sydney University's Glycemic Index Research Service.

ing of the drink mix for breakfast, your blood sugar levels and appetite would be stable for at least the next two hours.

Lunch

Lunch is a perfect time to take advantage of high-volume, low-calorie soups and salads. Adding PGX to the meal amplifies the volumetric and satiety effects of these foods. Or you can use the SlimStyles Weight Loss Drink Mix again as a meal replacement.

Dinner

For dinner, we want you to eat a healthy, balanced meal containing three or four food groups. Food choices should be voluminous and have a low-glycemic impact. Again we recommend you add PGX at dinner time to control overeating at night. And, if you find yourself hungry right after dinner, take an additional dosage of PGX to fight off the urge to eat.

RECIPE FOR A SUCCESSFUL MEAL

Create volume

To help you feel full, fill up on nonstarchy vegetables. These are considered "free" since they are high in fiber and very low in calories. Avoid large amounts or big portions of root vegetables, such as potatoes, parsnips, and squash, since these contain more starch and more calories.

Go for low-glycemic index foods

Choose fruit and starches that will not cause your blood sugar level to spike, and will take longer to digest and be absorbed in the bloodstream. These low GI foods will give your body better blood sugar control and sustained energy.

(continued on next page)

Aim for balance

When creating a balanced meal, include three or four food groups.

Lower the fat

- When cooking, try baking, broiling, grilling, poaching, roasting, sautéing with little oil, steaming, and stir-frying.
- Use nonstick cookware and use nonstick cooking sprays instead of butter, margarine, or oil to prepare foods with less or no fat.
- Skip gravy and rich sauces and enhance the flavor of foods by cooking with broth, stock, lemon juice, onions, and seasonings like garlic, ginger, cumin, spice blends, and herbs.
- Trim away any fat on meat and go skinless with poultry before cooking.

Reduce portion sizes

For more information on portion control, see chapter 5.

Snacks

Snacking is a very good habit as long as you keep the portion size small and calorie count low. You are allowed up to three snacks per day to be eaten between breakfast and lunch, lunch and dinner, and after dinner, if genuinely hungry. Snacks are a good way to keep your metabolism running throughout the day. However, unhealthy high-fat or -sugar snack choices lead to weight gain.

Choose snacks that contain a lot of nutrients and fiber, and make sure your snacks contain both carbohydrates and a source of protein. The carbohydrates provide you with some energy and the fiber and protein help make the energy last longer, keeping you full longer. The combination helps to maintain a slow rise and prevents a spike and quick fall in blood sugars. An easy way to remember this is that your snacks should contain two food groups.

Watch portion sizes. Aim for 100 to 150 calories per snack. That said, 150 calories from a chocolate bar or donut is not a healthy op-

TIPS FOR EATING HEALTHY WHEN YOU DON'T HAVE TIME TO COOK A MEAL

When you don't have time to prepare a meal or are preparing different foods for your family to eat, it's all right to have healthy convenience foods; just make sure that you add PGX to your meal.

Tip #1

Look for frozen entrees that are less than 350 calories and contain less than 10 grams of fat. Add a garden salad, vegetables, and fruit, to your healthy frozen entrees for a balanced meal. We like frozen entrees from companies such as Kashi, Seeds of Change, Helen's Kitchen, Amy's, and Sol Cuisine. Or on occasion you can choose some of the mainstream frozen entrees, such as those from Healthy Choice, Weight Watchers, Stouffer's Lean Cuisine Selections, Stouffer's Lean Cuisine Spa, South Beach Diet Entrees from Kraft, Michelina's Advantage, and Michelina's Lifestyle.

Tip #2

Having healthy frozen meats available to bake or grill is an easy way to get your protein. Some ideas include: salmon fillets; Atlantic cod; vegetarian patties; extra lean beef, turkey, chicken, or tuna; lemon-herb chicken breast; and chicken skewers. Also keeping frozen vegetables available can add volume, vitamins, and minerals to make a meal in a snap.

Tip #3

Prepare meals ahead of time. There is usually more time on the weekend to cook and enjoy meals with family and friends. Get a head start on busy weekday meals by making some meals ahead of time or making double batches of some recipes and freezing them for another day.

tion, since it only provides fat and sugar. Instead, choose healthy foods like an apple and 1 ounce low-fat cheese, an orange and small 100 grams container of low-fat yogurt, or six whole wheat crackers and 1 tablespoon of peanut butter.

FREE FOODS

Some vegetables are termed "free foods" and can be eaten in any desired amount because the calories they contain are offset by the number of calories your body burns in the process of digestion. If you are trying to lose weight, these foods are especially valuable as they can help to keep you feeling satisfied between meals. Consider the following vegetables as free foods that may be consumed in any amount and as often as desired in their raw form:

Alfalfa sprouts	Chinese cabbage	Radishes
Bell peppers	Cucumber	Spinach
Bok choy	Endive	Turnips
Cabbage	Escarole	Watercress
Chicory	Lettuce	
Celery	Parsley	

SNACKS CONTAINING 50 TO 100 CALORIES

GRAINS AND BREAD	Unit	Grams	Calories
Bread, 100% whole wheat, thin slice	1 piece	33	92
Crackers, rye, Norwegian flatbread	2 pieces	17	62
Crackers, 100% whole wheat	4 pieces	16	71
English muffin, 100% whole wheat	½ each	30	65
Graham crackers	2 pieces	14	59
Melba toast crackers, plain	3 pieces	15	59
Oatmeal, plain, instant	1 package	177	97
Popcorn, air-popped	2 cups	16	62

	Unit	Grams	Calories
Pumpernickel, thin slice	1 piece	20	50
Pita, 100% whole wheat	½ each	21	60
Tortilla, whole wheat	1 each	35	73
Whole wheat, 100%, thin slice	1 piece	33	92

DAIRY	Unit	Grams	Calories
Cottage cheese, 1%	⅓ cup	75	54
Cream cheese, low-fat	1½ tablespoons	23	52
Frozen yogurt, low-fat, chocolate	¼ cup	48	55
Frozen yogurt, low-fat, vanilla or strawberry	¼ cup	48	51
Milk, nonfat/skim	¾ cup	186	68
Mozzarella, low moisture, part skim	1-inch cube	18	53
Soy milk, plain or low-fat vanilla or chocolate	½ cup	123	60
Yogurt, fruit, nonfat	¼ cup	61	58

MEAT AND ALTERNATIVES	Unit	Grams	Calories
Eggs, hard-boiled	1 med	44	68
Nuts, almonds, whole	8 each	10	55
Nuts, peanuts, dry roasted, unsalted	9 each	9	53
Nuts, soy	15 grams	15	63
Nuts, walnuts	4 halves pieces	8	53
Salmon, pink, drained water-packed canned	1 can	56	76
Tuna, chunk white, drained water-packed canned	½ can	43	54

MEDIUM- AND LOW-GLYCEMIC INDEX FRUIT	Unit	Grams	Calories
Apples, fresh, chopped	1 cup	125	65
Apples, small	1 each	106	55

(continued on next page)

(continued from previous page)

MEDIUM- AND LOW-GLYCEMIC INDEX FRUIT	Unit	Grams	Calories
Applesauce, unsweetened	½ cup	122	52
Apricots, fresh	2 each	103	51
Banana, medium	½ each	59	53
Blueberries	¾ cup	109	62
Cherries, fresh	14 each	95	60
Grapefruit, fresh, small, red	1 each	200	64
Grapes, Thompson seedless, fresh	15 each	75	52
Kiwi, fresh, medium, without skin	2 each	152	92
Mandarin oranges, fresh, medium	2 each	168	90
Oranges, fresh, small	2 each	192	90
Peaches, fresh, medium	2 each	196	80
Pears, Bartlett, fresh, medium	1 each	166	96
Plums, fresh, medium	2 each	152	80
Strawberries	14 each	168	54
Tomatoes, fresh, red, cherry	18 each	306	55

DIPS	Unit	Grams	Calories
Babaganoush	1 tablespoon	14	70
Hummus	2 tablespoons	31	52
Salad dressing, Italian, reduced-fat	3 tablespoons	48	60
Salad dressing, Ranch, reduced-fat	2 tablespoons	30	65

FOUR-DAY SAMPLE MENU WITH SHOPPING LIST AND RECIPES

To help you get started in planning out your own daily menus, we are providing you with a four-day program complete with menus and recipes. Since most people do not have the time to get to the grocery store every day, we wanted to show you how to shop for a four-day period.

By following this program a couple of times, you can get in the habit of planning out your meals well in advance and replenishing your perishables every three to four days.

Because we have been frustrated by cookbooks designed for healthier eating that were packed full of difficult (or nearly impossible to get) ingredients, and recipes that took too long to prepare or required too many steps to prepare, we have chosen recipes that can be prepared and cooked within thirty minutes or less. We have also chosen recipes that have a short list of ingredients or readily available ingredients with no difficult steps to follow. We hope you find them as easy and enjoyable as we do. For more tested recipes that can easily be modified to create a healthier version, go to www.recipezaar.com.

Menus
Day 1
Breakfast
  SlimStyles Weight Loss Drink Mix

Midmorning snack
  1 medium orange

Lunch
  Field Greens Salad with Healthy Oil Dressing (page 193)
  Red Bean and Tomato Soup (page 194)
  Ry-Vita or Wasa whole-grain rye crackers

Midafternoon snack
  6 celery sticks, 4 inches in length

Dinner
  Field Greens Salad with Bell peppers, Carrots, and Radishes
    (page 194)
  Minted Carrots with Pumpkin Seeds (page 195)
  Steamed Broccoli (page 195)
  Asian Salmon (page 195)
  Whole-grain bread or roll
  Fresh Raspberries (page 196)

Evening tea
  1 or 2 cups of herbal tea (no caffeine)

Day 2

Breakfast
  SlimStyles Weight Loss Drink Mix

Midmorning snack
  2 tablespoons almonds
  ½ cup blueberries

Lunch
  Tuna Salad Wrap (page 196)

Midafternoon snack
  1 medium red pear

Dinner
  Jicama Salad (page 197)
  Black Bean Chili (page 198)
  Whole-wheat tortillas
  Diced Pineapple (page 198)

Evening tea
  1 or 2 cups of herbal tea (no caffeine)

Day 3

Breakfast
  SlimStyles Weight Loss Drink Mix

Midmorning snack
  ½ cup blueberries
  2 tablespoons almonds

Lunch
  Italian White Bean Soup (page 199)

Midafternoon snack
  1 medium red pear

Dinner
  Orange and Fennel Salad (page 200)
  Curried Tofu over Brown Rice (page 200)
  Dr. Murray's Favorite Greens (page 201)
  Blueberries (page 201)

Evening tea
  1 or 2 cups of herbal tea (no caffeine)

Day 4
Breakfast
  SlimStyles Weight Loss Drink Mix

Midmorning snack
  1 medium red apple

Lunch
  Black Bean Salad (page 202)

Midafternoon snack
  16 carrot sticks, 4 inches in length

Dinner
  Mediterranean Salad (page 202)
  Quick Acorn Squash (page 203)
  Polenta Puttanesca with Tofu (page 203)
  Fresh Mango Slices (page 204)

Evening tea
  1 cup herbal tea (no caffeine)

Recipes
The recipes we are providing allow for substitutions and modifications based upon your own tastes; just try not to alter the caloric content too

much in doing so. For example, if a recipe contains a vegetable that you do not like, substitute one you do like. The recipes are based on providing two servings. You can adjust the number of servings up or down as needed. For example, for four servings simply double the recipe.

Shopping list

The following shopping list represents the items needed for the complete four-day menu: We recommend buying organic whenever possible.

PGX

SlimStyles Weight Loss Drink Mix—1 jar each of at least 2 flavors for variety
PGX Granules—1 jar
PGX SlimStyx—1 box
PGX soft gel capsules—1 bottle

HERBAL TEA

Most of the major brands of herbal tea—Celestial Seasons, Bigelow, Republic of Tea, Traditional Medicinals—provide a sampler pack to help you identify teas that appeal to you. Try to choose decaffeinated varieties, especially with your nighttime cup of tea. If you feel you need a little caffeine in the morning, go with a cup of regular green tea. In general, avoid black teas.

PRODUCE

Try to buy organic, if possible, and be sure to wash all produce before consumption.

Acorn squash—1
Basil—1 bunch
Bell peppers—3 green; 2 red
Blueberries—1 pint
Broccoli—2 heads
Cabbage—½ head, green or red
Carrots—One 1-pound bag

Celery—2 bunches
Cilantro—1 bunch
Cucumber—2 medium-sized
Fennel—1 small bulb
Garlic—2 heads
Ginger—2 inches fresh

Green onions (scallions)—
1 bunch
Jicama—1
Kale—2 large bunches
Lemons—4
Mango—1
Mint (fresh)—1 small bunch
Mixed field greens—10- to
12-ounce bag
Mushrooms—5-ounce package
Onions—4
Oranges—4

Parsley (fresh)—1 bunch
Pear—2 red
Plums—4 medium
Radishes—1 bunch
Raspberries—½ pint
Red or green grapes—½ pound
Romaine lettuce—1 head
Shiitake mushrooms—4 ounces
Tomatoes, fresh—6 medium
Tomatoes, Roma or plum—
2 medium
Tomatoes, cherry—½ pint

FISH AND POULTRY

Chicken breast—1 boneless,
skinless (8 ounces)
Salmon—½ pound fresh
fillet

Tuna—1 6-ounce can
(or 7-ounce foil pouch)
low-sodium, chunk
white in spring water

MISCELLANEOUS GROCERY ITEMS

Balsamic vinegar—1 bottle
Dijon mustard—8-ounce jar
Honey (raw)—8-ounce jar
Kalamata olives—1 small jar
Soy milk, nonfat milk, or
nonfat yogurt—1 quart
Tofu—one 15-ounce
container, firm
Whey protein (vanilla for sure
and any other flavors to

suit your palate)—
16 ounces. (NOTE: We
recommend Whey Factors
from Natural Factors
because it contains no
added sugar or
additives.)
Coconut milk—
14-ounce can

NUTS, SEEDS, AND DRIED FRUIT

Almonds (raw)—1 cup shelled
(5 ounces)
Walnuts (raw)—1 cup shelled
(4 ounces)

Pumpkin seeds—½ cup
shelled

Oils
Flaxseed oil—1 bottle, 12 to 16 ounces
Olive oil (extra virgin) or macadamia nut oil—1 bottle, 12 to 16 ounces

Grains and Pasta
Brown rice (quick)—1 box
  (1 pound)
Polenta (quick)—1 box (375 g)
Rolled oats—1 small container
  (18 ounces)

Ry-Vita or Wasa whole-grain
  rye crackers—1 package
Whole-grain rolls—2
Whole-wheat tortillas—
  1 package of 8 or 10

Frozen Foods
Corn (frozen)—10-ounce
  package

Canned Foods
Chicken or vegetable broth—
  six 11- to 14-ounce cans
Beans, chickpeas—
  15-ounce can
Beans, red kidney—three
  15-ounce cans
Beans, black beans—
  15-ounce can

Beans, white—15-ounce can
Tomatoes, diced—
  14.5-ounce can
Tomato sauce—two 8-ounce
  cans low-sodium
Tomato soup, low-sodium—
  10.75-ounce can

Spices and Seasonings
Italian herbs (seasoning)
Allspice or nutmeg, ground
Balsamic vinegar
Capers (in a jar with salt
  and vinegar)
Chili powder
Cinnamon, ground
Crushed red pepper flakes
Cumin, ground

Curry powder
Ginger (dried)
Ground black pepper
No Salt, Nu-Salt, or Also Salt—
  potassium chloride salts to
  use as a substitute for regu-
  lar salt (sodium chloride)
Soy sauce (low-sodium)
Thyme

RECIPES FOR DAY 1

BREAKFAST
SlimStyles Weight Loss Drink Mix

MIDMORNING SNACK
1 medium orange

LUNCH

Field Greens Salad with Healthy Oil Dressing
2 SERVINGS SALAD, 24 SERVINGS DRESSING (1 ¼ CUPS)

Most supermarkets and grocery stores now have mixed field greens in the produce section or in pre-packaged plastic bags. This convenience makes a simple mixed field green salad a perfect quick and easy salad.

HEALTHY OIL DRESSING
½ cup olive or macadamia nut oil
½ cup flaxseed oil
2 tablespoons fresh lemon juice
2 tablespoons balsamic vinegar
2 garlic cloves, finely minced
1 tablespoon Italian herbs
1 teaspoon salt substitute
1 teaspoon pepper

4 cups mixed field greens

Place all the ingredients except the greens in a blender and blend for 2 to 3 minutes until emulsified. Store in a tightly closed jar in your refrigerator for a quick and easy, health-promoting salad dressing. Use no more than 1 tablespoon daily.

To serve, toss the greens to coat with 2 tablespoons dressing and divide between two plates.

Red Bean and Tomato Soup

2 SERVINGS

½ cup chopped onion
1 clove garlic, chopped
1 stalk celery, chopped
1 tablespoon olive oil
1 cup canned red kidney beans, drained
One 10.75-can low-sodium tomato soup
2 tablespoons Italian herbs
Salt substitute and pepper to taste
2 Ry-Vita or Wasa whole-grain rye crackers

Sauté the onions, garlic, and celery in olive oil over medium-low heat for about 5 minutes in a medium saucepan, stirring often. Blend the kidney beans, tomato soup, and herbs in a blender for 2 to 3 minutes. Add to the pot along with one cup of water. Cook for 15 minutes. Season to taste. Serve with one cracker each.

MIDAFTERNOON SNACK
6 celery sticks, 4 inches in length

DINNER

Field Greens Salad with Bell Peppers, Carrots, and Radishes

2 SERVINGS

4 cups mixed field greens
1 green bell pepper, chopped
½ cup chopped carrots
½ cup chopped radishes
2 tablespoons Healthy Oil Dressing (page 193)

Toss all ingredients in a large bowl. Your serving size should be about two cups.

Minted Carrots with Pumpkin Seeds

2 SERVINGS

3 medium carrots, peeled and cut into rounds
1 tablespoon chopped fresh parsley
1 tablespoon chopped fresh mint
2 tablespoons coarsely chopped pumpkin seeds
1 tablespoon fresh lemon juice
1 tablespoon olive oil
Salt substitute and pepper

Steam the carrots until still slightly crunchy. Toss in a medium bowl with the parsley, mint, pumpkin seeds, lemon juice, oil, and salt substitute and pepper to taste.

Steamed Broccoli

2 SERVINGS

½ head broccoli

Separate the florets and cut the stalks into pieces. Steam in a covered saucepan until bright green but still crunchy.

Asian Salmon

2 SERVINGS

2 teaspoons low-sodium soy sauce
1 tablespoon Dijon mustard
½ pound salmon fillet, skinned and cut into 2 pieces
½ cup sliced onion
1 clove garlic, chopped
¼ teaspoon dried ginger (or 1½ teaspoons minced fresh ginger)
2 cups sliced fresh shiitake mushrooms

Preheat the oven to 375°F. Mix the soy sauce into the mustard and coat salmon. Sauté the onion, garlic, ginger, and mushrooms in a medium skillet for about 5 minutes. Bake the salmon in a baking dish, depending on how thick it is (about 7 minutes if less than an inch thick). When cooked, place on a bed of sautéed mushrooms.

Fresh Raspberries

2 SERVINGS

1 cup fresh raspberries
Vanilla soy milk or nonfat yogurt, optional

Served chilled in a ½-cup serving size. Add little soy milk or yogurt, if desired.

RECIPES FOR DAY 2

BREAKFAST
SlimStyles Weight Loss Drink Mix

MIDMORNING SNACK
2 tablespoons almonds
½ cup blueberries

LUNCH

Tuna Salad Wrap

2 SERVINGS

1 6-ounce or 7-ounce foil pouch low-sodium
   chunk white tuna in spring water
¼ cup minced onion
1 stalk celery, chopped
1 teaspoon fresh lemon juice
1 tablespoon olive oil
1 tablespoon chopped fresh parsley
2 tablespoons Dijon mustard
½ teaspoon salt substitute
½ teaspoon pepper
2 whole-wheat tortillas or 2 slices whole-grain bread

Mix all the ingredients except the tortillas in a bowl. Spoon onto the tortillas and wrap. Whole-grain bread may be substituted to make open-face sandwiches.

MIDAFTERNOON SNACK
2 medium plums

DINNER

Jicama Salad

2 SERVINGS

1 cup julienned peeled jicama
1 orange, peeled, sectioned, and cut into chunks
1 medium cucumber, seeded and thinly sliced
¼ cup chopped green onions (scallions)
¼ cup chopped fresh cilantro
1 tablespoon chopped fresh mint
¼ cup fresh orange juice
¼ cup fresh lemon or lime juice
¼ teaspoon salt substitute
¼ teaspoon pepper
¼ teaspoon chili powder

Combine the jicama, orange, cucumber, onion, cilantro, and mint in a large bowl. In another bowl, mix the orange juice, lemon juice, salt substitute, pepper, and chili powder. Pour the juice mixture over jicama mixture, and toss gently. Cover and chill for at least 20 minutes before serving.

Black Bean Chili

2 SERVINGS

½ medium onion, chopped
2 cloves garlic, chopped
1 green bell pepper, diced
1 tablespoon olive oil
1 cup chicken or light vegetable broth
One 15-ounce can black beans, drained
1 cup frozen corn kernels
½ cup low-sodium tomato sauce
1 tablespoon ground cumin
1 tablespoon chili powder
1 tablespoon Italian herbs
½ teaspoon salt substitute
½ teaspoon pepper
¼ cup chopped fresh cilantro
2 whole-wheat tortillas

Sauté onion, garlic, and green pepper in olive oil in a medium sauce-pan over medium-low heat for about 5 minutes, stirring frequently. Add the chicken broth, beans, corn, tomato sauce, cumin, chili pow-der, herbs, salt substitute, and pepper and simmer for 15 minutes. Add the cilantro as garnish and season with additional salt substitute and pepper if needed. Serve with heated whole-wheat tortillas.

Diced Pineapple

Peel and core a whole pineapple and cut into bite-sized pieces. Place half of the pineapple in the refrigerator for your midmorning snack the next day and serve the other half for dessert.

RECIPES FOR DAY 3

BREAKFAST
SlimStyles Weight Loss Drink Mix

MIDMORNING SNACK

¼ pineapple with ½ cup blueberries

2 tablespoon almonds

LUNCH

Italian White Bean Soup

2 SERVINGS

½ onion thinly sliced
1 tablespoon olive oil
4 cloves garlic, sliced
2 cups chicken or light vegetable broth
2 cups finely chopped collard greens or kale (cut out stem first)
1 cup canned diced tomatoes
2 teaspoons Italian herbs
One 15-ounce can navy or small white beans, drained
Salt substitute and pepper

Sauté the onion in olive oil in a medium saucepan over medium-low heat for 5 minutes, stirring frequently. Add the garlic and continue to sauté for another minute. Add the broth, greens, tomatoes, and herbs. Simmer for 15 minutes over medium heat. Add the beans and cook for another 5 minutes. Season to taste.

MIDAFTERNOON SNACK

1 medium red pear

DINNER

Orange and Fennel Salad

2 SERVINGS

1 orange
1 small bulb fennel
1 small head romaine lettuce, cut up
¼ cup chopped fresh parsley
1 tablespoon Healthy Oil Dressing (page 193)

Remove the peel and white pith from the orange. Slice the orange and fennel, then toss with greens and dressing in a large bowl.

Curried Tofu over Brown Rice

2 SERVINGS

½ cup uncooked quick brown rice
7½ ounces firm tofu or 1 boneless, skinless chicken breast half
½ cup chopped onion
Olive oil
1 clove garlic, minced
½ teaspoon powdered ginger
2 teaspoons curry powder
1 cup chicken or vegetable broth
1 medium red bell pepper, chopped
½ cup coconut milk (make sure it is mixed well before measuring)
Salt substitute and pepper

Follow the instructions on the package of quick brown rice. While the water for the rice is coming to a boil, cut the tofu or chicken into small cubes. Sauté the onion in a little olive oil in a medium skillet over medium-low heat for about 5 minutes, stirring frequently. Add the garlic and ginger and continue to sauté for another minute, then remove from heat and add the curry powder. Mix well. Return to the heat and add broth, tofu, bell pepper, and coconut milk. Simmer until tofu or chicken is done, about 10 minutes. Season to taste.

Place the rice on a plate and top with the curry.

Dr. Murray's Favorite Greens

2 SERVINGS

1 tablespoon olive oil
1 teaspoon balsamic vinegar
1 large bunch kale, washed, trimmed, and coarsely chopped
½ cup diced green onion (scallions)
1 clove garlic, thinly sliced
½ cup coarsely chopped walnuts or almonds
¼ teaspoon salt substitute
½ teaspoon black pepper
Lemon wedges

Heat the olive oil and balsamic vinegar in large skillet or wok over medium-high heat. Add the kale, onions, garlic, and walnuts, and sauté until soft. Season with the salt substitute and pepper. Serve with lemon wedges.

Blueberries

2 SERVINGS

1 cup fresh blueberries
Vanilla soy milk or nonfat yogurt, optional

Served chilled in a ½-cup serving size. Add a little vanilla soy milk or nonfat yogurt, if desired.

RECIPES FOR DAY 4

BREAKFAST
SlimStyles Weight Loss Drink Mix

MIDMORNING SNACK
1 medium red apple

Black Bean Salad

2 SERVINGS

One 15-ounce can black beans, drained and rinsed
1 cup frozen corn, thawed
6 cherry tomatoes, quartered
½ cup minced green onion (scallion)
1 clove garlic, pressed
½ cup diced red bell pepper
½ cup chopped cilantro
2 cups mixed field greens
1 tablespoon olive or flaxseed oil
2 tablespoons fresh lemon juice
¼ cup chopped cilantro
Salt substitute and pepper

Mix all ingredients together in a large bowl and serve.

MIDAFTERNOON SNACK
6 carrot sticks, 4 inches in length

DINNER

Mediterranean Salad

2 SERVINGS

1 cup chopped fresh tomato (cut out excess flesh if pulpy)
1 cup chopped peeled cucumber
½ cup finely minced green onion (scallion)
1 clove garlic, finely minced
1 cup canned chickpeas, drained and rinsed
1 tablespoon fresh lemon juice
1 tablespoon chopped fresh parsley
1 teaspoon Italian herbs
1 tablespoon olive oil

Mix all ingredients together in a large bowl and chill for at least 15 minutes.

Quick Acorn Squash

2 SERVINGS

1 acorn squash, cut in half, seeds removed
1 tablespoon honey
Dash of ground cinnamon

Place the squash in a microwave-safe dish with cut side up. Cover and cook in the microwave for 10 to 13 minutes on HIGH or until fork tender. Top with the honey and cinnamon.

Polenta Puttanesca with Tofu

2 SERVINGS

SAUCE
1 onion, diced
1 clove garlic, crushed or minced
Olive oil
1 green bell pepper, diced
1½ cups tomato sauce
7½ ounces firm tofu, cut into small cubes
1 tablespoon Italian herbs
1 bay leaf
1 teaspoon crushed red pepper flakes
2 tablespoons capers, rinsed and drained
4 to 6 pitted Kalamata olives, coarsely chopped
1 tablespoon finely chopped fresh parsley
¼ teaspoon salt substitute
½ teaspoon pepper

POLENTA
1 cup instant polenta (adjust water amount if needed as per package
    instructions)
1 teaspoon salt substitute

For the sauce: In a large saucepan, sauté the onion and garlic in a little oil over medium heat for 3 to 4 minutes. Add peppers and sauté for 3 to 4 more minutes. Add 1 cup water and bring to a boil. Cover pot and simmer for 15 minutes. Add the tomato sauce, tofu, herbs, bay leaf, red pepper, capers, olives, parsley, salt substitute, and pepper, and simmer for another hour, stirring occasionally. Remove from the heat, remove the bay leaf, and allow to cool slightly before pouring over polenta.

For the polenta: Bring 3 cups water to a boil in a 2-quart saucepan. Add the salt substitute and reduce heat until water is simmering. Add the polenta very slowly. To avoid lumps, stir quickly with a long-handled spoon while adding the polenta. Cook, stirring continuously 5 minutes or until mixture is solid, but still soft. Pour into large bowls or plates. Let cool about 10 minutes, or until firm, before pouring on the sauce.

Fresh Mango Slices

2 SERVINGS

1 fresh mango, peeled and pitted

Slice up the mango for a refreshing desert.

CHAPTER SUMMARY

- Long-term weight loss success is based upon achieving five key goals:
  - Effectively decrease appetite, leading to a reduction of calories consumed
  - Normalize and stabilize blood glucose levels
  - Increase metabolism and the burning of fat, while preserving lean muscle mass
  - Reset the mechanisms that control individual fat cell size and body weight
  - Make food and lifestyle choices that promote ideal body weight and create a healthier relationship with food
- We recommend creating a journal to record a detailed account of your feelings, thoughts, and emotions as you embark on the Hunger Free Forever program.
- The key ingredient to successful weight loss is the ingestion of 2.5

to 5 grams of PGX at major meals and perhaps at least twice more for those with an appetite more difficult to tame.

- The best breakfast that we can recommend for effective weight loss or management is the SlimStyles Weight Loss Drink mix.
- Lunch is a perfect time to take advantage of high-volume, low-calorie soups and salads.
- For dinner, eat a healthy, balanced meal containing three to four food groups. Food choices should be voluminous and have a low-glycemic impact.
- Snacks are a good way to keep your metabolism running throughout the day; however, unhealthy snacks or high-fat or -sugar snack choices lead to weight gain.

11

ADDITIONAL RECIPES
FOR HIGH SATIETY

In order to help you to eat for high satiety to achieve and maintain your ideal body weight, in this chapter we are providing a variety of additional recipes to help you follow a low-glycemic load diet, increase your intake dietary fiber, support liver function and diet-induced thermogenesis, and prevent sarcopenia and build muscle mass. These recipes are easy to prepare, easy to follow, and taste great. Remember, you can modify or substitute a recipe based upon your own tastes; just try not to alter the caloric content too much in doing so. With the exception of the breakfast recipes, which are based upon single servings, these recipes all provide two servings. You can adjust the number of servings up or down as needed.

If you have some recipes of your own that you would like to make healthier, here are some suggestions: substitute Egg Beaters or egg whites for whole eggs (see facing page for conversion chart); substitute butter with macadamia nut oil or coconut oil; use nonfat dairy versus whole-fat forms, especially for items such as sour cream, cream cheese, and yogurt; and most important adjust the portion size of the serving to provide the caloric goal for the dish.

BREAKFAST RECIPES

As a reminder, we feel that the SlimStyles Weight Loss Drink Mix is a great way to start the day. It comes in a variety of flavors and you can always add a half cup of frozen berries or other fruit to make it even more satisfying. But we recognize that a change of pace is often desired. Healthy, satisfying breakfasts are easy to prepare. The recipes following are based on providing one serving, you can adjust the number of servings up or down as needed (e.g., for two servings simply double the recipe). You will notice that we recommend alternative sweeteners in a couple of these recipes. For a complete guide to sugar substitutes, see appendix C.

EGG SUBSTITUTES

Egg substitutes like Egg Beaters are composed of egg whites. You can also now buy pure egg whites as well. Egg whites are an exceptional protein and a very easy, low-calorie way to boost protein levels. Egg Beaters and other egg white products can be used in place of whole eggs in all of your favorite recipes. Here is the conversion chart for egg substitutes like Egg Beaters:

¼ cup egg substitute = 1 egg

2 tablespoons egg substitute = 1 egg white

3 tablespoons egg substitute = 1 egg yolk

Nutritional comparison

	½ cup Egg Beaters	2 eggs
Calories	60	150
Total fat	0	10 g
Cholesterol	0	420 mg
Carbohydrates	2 g	2 g
Protein	12 g	12 g

Whey-Enhanced Instant Oatmeal with PGX

1 SERVING

⅓ cup instant oatmeal
25 grams whey protein (vanilla or unflavored)
2 teaspoons xylitol (or natural stevia-based sweetener to taste)
2.5 to 5 grams PGX
1 teaspoon ground cinnamon

Bring 1½ cups of water to a boil. In a bowl, mix the oatmeal, whey protein, sweetener, PGX, and cinnamon. Add the water gradually to the bowl, stirring vigorously with a whisk or fork.

Happy Apple Cinnamon Oat n' PGX

1 SERVING

½ cup diced unpeeled golden delicious apples
⅛ teaspoon salt substitute
½ teaspoon ground cinnamon
¼ teaspoon ground nutmeg
⅓ cup uncooked old-fashioned oats
2 teaspoons xylitol (or natural stevia-based sweetener to taste)
Nonfat milk, optional

Combine the apples, ⅓ cup water, salt if using, cinnamon, and nutmeg in a small saucepan. Bring to a boil. Stir in the oats, reduce the heat, and cook about 7 minutes. Serve with xylitol, and nonfat milk if desired.

Simple Egg Substitute or Egg White Omelet

1 SERVING

3 egg whites or ¾ cup egg substitute
1 tablespoon sliced green onions (scallions)
2 tablespoons diced green or red bell pepper
1½ teaspoons olive oil, or olive oil cooking spray
⅛ teaspoon pepper
⅛ teaspoon salt substitute
1 tablespoon shredded low-fat Cheddar cheese

Whisk the egg whites in a small bowl to blend. Add the green onions and bell pepper. Heat the olive oil in a small skillet (or spray with cooking spray) over medium heat. Pour in the egg mixture. Add the salt and pepper. Cover and cook for about 4 minutes, until almost set (sprinkle with the cheese and replace the cover. Cook for 30 to 45 seconds until cheese is melted.

Mediterranean Omelet

1 SERVING

1 ½ teaspoons olive oil
½ clove garlic, minced
¼ red bell pepper, cut in ½-inch dice
2 tablespoons diced onions
1 tablespoon minced sun-dried tomatoes (packed in oil, drained)
⅓ cup egg substitute
1 tablespoon shredded mozzarella cheese

Heat a small nonstick skillet over medium heat. Add the olive oil, garlic, bell pepper, and onion, and cooking until softened. Add the tomatoes, then pour in the egg substitute and rotate pan to distribute evenly. Lift the edges of the omelet, tilting the pan to allow the liquid to run under the cooked egg substitute. Lower the heat to medium-low and cook, without stirring until set. Sprinkle the cheese on one half of omelet, then fold over, enclosing the cheese.

SOUP RECIPES

The recipes following are exceptionally nutritious and a great way to start off a meal. We also think soup can be a fantastic meal alone, especially the heartier versions that we provide recipes for here.

Tuscan White Bean and Spinach Soup

2 SERVINGS

½ shallot, finely diced
½ clove garlic, minced
1 teaspoon olive oil
1½ to 2 cups fat free chicken or vegetable broth
One 7.5-ounce can diced tomatoes, with juice
One 7.5-ounce (or ½ 15-ounce) can white beans (cannelloni or other)
½ teaspoon dried rosemary
Salt substitute and pepper
Crushed red pepper flakes
1½ cups packed cleaned and trimmed baby spinach

In a large saucepan, sauté the shallot and garlic in the olive oil. Add the broth, tomatoes, beans, and rosemary. Season as desired with salt substitute, pepper, and red pepper flakes. Bring to a boil, reduce heat and let simmer for 2 minutes. If the soup seems too thick for your liking add a bit more broth. Add the spinach and cook until wilted.

Recipe modified from original, courtesy of www.recipezaar.com.

Lebanese Chicken Stew

2 SERVINGS

Olive oil
8 ounces boneless, skinless chicken breast, cubed
1 very small leek, white part only, thinly sliced
1 medium clove garlic, crushed
1 teaspoon grated fresh ginger
1 small red onion, peeled and quartered
¼ teaspoon saffron threads
¼ teaspoon ground cinnamon
¼ teaspoon ground ginger
¾ cup chicken broth
1 small tomato, seeded and diced
1 dried date, seeded and minced
1 tablespoon fresh lemon juice
Salt substitute and pepper

Heat 2 teaspoons olive oil in medium saucepan and brown the chicken. Set aside. Add a little more oil and gently sauté the leek, garlic, ginger, and onion until softened, 5 to 8 minutes. Add the saffron, cinnamon, ginger, and broth. Cover the pot and simmer for 20 minutes or so, until the mixture has turned a beautiful saffron yellow. Return the chicken to the pot along with the tomato and date and simmer for 30 to 40 minutes until the chicken is tender. Add the lemon juice. Season to taste.

Recipe modified from original, courtesy of www.recipezaar.com.

Kidney Bean, Barley, and Sweet Potato Stew

2 SERVINGS

1 cup vegetable broth
2 tablespoons pearl barley
1 cup canned kidney beans, rinsed and drained
¼ large onion, diced
1 small sweet potato, peeled and diced
1 small stalk celery, diced
⅛ teaspoon pepper
¼ teaspoon salt substitute
⅛ teaspoon dried thyme, crushed
¼ teaspoon dried sage

In a medium saucepan, bring the broth to a boil. Stir in the barley, reduce the heat, and cover. Simmer for 30 minutes, stirring occasionally. Add the beans, onion, sweet potato, celery, pepper, salt substitute, thyme, and sage, and simmer, covered, for 20 minutes or until the vegetables are tender. Stir occasionally, and add broth if the stew dries out.

Tomato and Turkey Soup

2 SERVINGS

1 cup chicken broth
One 14-ounce diced tomatoes
1 tablespoon tomato puree or tomato paste
½ cup instant brown rice
1 clove garlic, minced
¼ teaspoon caraway seeds
8 ounces extra-lean ground turkey breast
⅛ teaspoon pepper
⅛ teaspoon salt substitute
1 tablespoon freshly chopped basil

Put the broth, tomatoes, and tomato puree into a large heavy saucepan and bring to a boil. Add the rice, stirring briskly for about 5 minutes, then reduce the heat to a simmer. While the rice and tomatoes are cooking, in a mixing bowl combine the garlic, caraway seeds, turkey, salt substitute, and pepper. Mix together well. Shape into 16 small balls. Carefully drop them into the tomato stock and simmer for 8 to 10 minutes, until the turkey balls and rice are cooked. Garnish with chopped basil.

Turkish Red Lentil Soup

2 SERVINGS

1 cup red lentils, washed and cleaned
1 quart vegetable broth
½ cup peeled and diced white potatoes (1 small)
¼ cup finely chopped mild onions
1 teaspoon paprika
Salt substitute and pepper

Place the red lentils in a colander and rinse. Sift through to remove debris or damaged beans. Place the washed and cleaned lentils into a medium saucepan with the broth, potatoes, onions, and paprika. Bring the pot to a boil and reduce to a simmer. Loosely place a lid on the pot. Cook for 40 to 45 minutes until the lentils are tender. Then, place all but 1 cup of the soup into a blender or food processor and blend briefly. Return blended soup to the pot with the reserved cup of soup. Heat through. Add salt substitute and pepper to taste.

Recipe modified from original, courtesy of www.recipezaar.com.

Creamy Chickpea & Rosemary Soup

2 SERVINGS

1 tablespoon olive oil
2 cloves garlic, finely chopped
½ tablespoon minced fresh rosemary leaves, plus sprigs for garnish
½ teaspoon crushed red pepper flakes
One (15- to 19-ounce) can chickpeas, rinsed and drained
2 cups chicken or vegetable broth
1 tablespoon fresh lemon juice
Salt substitute

In a large saucepan, heat the olive oil over medium heat and add garlic, rosemary, and red pepper flakes. Cook, stirring constantly, until the garlic starts to brown, about 1 minute. Add the chickpeas and cook 2 minutes, stirring constantly. Add the chicken broth and bring to a boil. Reduce the heat and simmer 30 minutes. Let the soup cool slightly, then transfer it to a blender. Puree until just smooth. Return to the saucepan, reheat, and stir in the lemon juice and salt substitute to taste. Serve garnished with fresh rosemary.

Recipe modified from original, courtesy of www.recipezaar.com.

Spicy Black Bean Soup

2 SERVINGS

1 tablespoon olive oil
1 medium onion, chopped
2 cloves garlic, minced
1 teaspoon dried thyme
One 15-ounce can black beans, rinsed and drained
2 cups chicken or vegetable broth
1 cup diced tomatoes (canned are okay)
1 teaspoon ground cumin
½ teaspoon Tabasco sauce

In a medium saucepan, heat the olive oil over medium heat. Add the onion and cook until the onion is soft and translucent. Add the garlic and thyme, cooking for 3 minutes more. Add the beans, broth, tomatoes, cumin, and Tabasco and bring to a boil. Reduce heat to medium-low, cover, and simmer for 20 to 30 minutes; stirring occasionally. Remove 3 cups of the soup from the pot and puree in a blender until smooth. Add the puree back to the soup and reheat until the soup is thoroughly warmed. Adjust with more Tabasco, if desired.

Recipe modified from original, courtesy of www.recipezaar.com.

Free Food Soup

2 SERVINGS

The serving size, about a quart, for this soup is very large, but the calorie content is quite low.

1 tablespoon olive oil
2 carrots, peeled and cut into 1-inch slices
2 stalks celery, sliced
1 large onion, chopped
1 clove garlic, minced
One 8-ounce can tomato sauce
½ medium head cauliflower, cut into bite-sized pieces
1 zucchini, cut into 1-inch chunks

One 5-ounce package spinach leaves, rinsed
½ cup chopped fresh parsley
1 quart chicken broth
½ teaspoon pepper
1 teaspoon salt substitute

In a large saucepan, heat the olive oil over medium heat. Add the carrots, celery, onion, and garlic. Cook, stirring occasionally, about 5 minutes. Stir in the tomato sauce. Add the cauliflower, zucchini, spinach, parsley, broth, pepper, and salt substitute. Bring to a boil over high heat, stirring occasionally. Reduce heat to low; cover and simmer, stirring occasionally, for 15 to 20 minutes or until the veggies are tender. Taste and add more salt substitute and pepper if needed.

Healthy Bean Soup with Kale

2 SERVINGS

1 tablespoon olive oil
2 cloves garlic, minced
½ medium yellow onion, chopped
2 cups chopped raw kale (remove stems first)
2 cups chicken or vegetable broth
One 7.5 ounce (or ½ 15-ounce) can cannellini or navy, or other white
    beans, undrained
One 7.5 ounce can diced tomatoes
1 teaspoon Italian herbs
⅛ teaspoon salt substitute
⅛ teaspoon pepper
½ cup chopped parsley

In a large saucepan, heat the olive oil. Add the garlic and onion; sauté until soft. Wash the kale, leaving small droplets of water. Add the kale to the pot and sauté until wilted, about 15 minutes. Add the broth, beans, tomatoes, herbs, salt substitute, and pepper. Cook until heated through. Garnish with the chopped parsley.

Recipe modified from original, courtesy of www.recipezaar.com.

White Chicken Chili

2 SERVINGS

8 ounces boneless, skinless chicken breasts, cubed
One 14.5-ounce can chicken broth
1 small onion, chopped
1 clove garlic, minced
½ of a 4-ounce can chopped green chiles
One 15-ounce can white beans, drained
½ teaspoon ground cumin
¼ teaspoon dried oregano
¼ teaspoon pepper
¼ teaspoon salt substitute
⅛ teaspoon cayenne pepper
⅓ bunch green onions (scallions), thinly sliced, for garnish

Sauté the chicken in a nonstick skillet until lightly browned; remove from the heat and set aside. Pour half of the chicken broth into a large saucepan and add onion and garlic. Bring to a simmer and cook until the onion starts to soften. Add the chiles, stir, then add the remaining broth and the beans. Stir in the cumin, oregano, black pepper, salt substitute, and cayenne. Bring to a boil and add the chicken. Cover and simmer for 30 to 45 minutes. Serve garnished with sliced green onion.

SALAD RECIPES

It is very important to have a salad with most meals. The more hearty salads, just like the heartier soups, can be meals on their own. The salad recipes following are listed in increasing order of calorie density. So, the later salads are designed to be entrees. Don't be afraid to create your own salads. Focus on salads that have a lot of vegetables and volume. Make liberal use of the "free foods" and be sure to use modest amounts of salad dressing, unless it is low calorie.

Basic Green Salad Equation

2 SERVINGS

2 to 4 cups chopped of one of the following or a mixture: romaine lettuce, iceberg lettuce, spinach, Boston or bibb lettuce, field greens, endive, arugula, escarole, watercress

1 or more cups of any combination of the following: alfalfa sprouts, diced bell pepper, fresh berries, diced or sliced carrots, diced or sliced cucumber, whole or torn fresh herbs, sliced mushrooms, whole or chopped parsley leaves, diced or sliced radishes, thinly sliced red onions, spinach leaves, whole or chopped strawberries, diced or sliced tomatoes, diced or sliced turnips, diced or sliced zucchini

Simply combine in a large bowl and toss.

Everything But the Kitchen Sink Thai Salad

2 SERVINGS

SALAD

1 small head romaine lettuce, chopped
1 red bell pepper, cut into strips
1 carrot, peeled and shredded
1⅓ cups bean sprouts
1 small cucumber, halved and sliced
⅔ cup trimmed and cut snow peas
¼ cup slivered red onions
⅓ cup chopped fresh cilantro
⅓ cup chopped fresh mint

DRESSING

2 tablespoons lime juice
1 tablespoon coconut oil
1 tablespoon sesame oil
2 teaspoons xylitol (or natural stevia-based sweetener to taste)
1 teaspoon soy sauce
1 clove garlic, minced
½ teaspoon cayenne pepper

Toss salad ingredients in a large bowl. In a small bowl, whisk dressing ingredients until xylitol is dissolved. Gently toss salad with dressing and serve.

Healthy Greek Salad

2 SERVINGS

½ red bell pepper, seeded and cut into 1-inch chunks
¼ green bell pepper, seeded and cut into 1-inch chunks
½ cup cherry tomatoes (cut half in half; leave the rest whole)
½ cucumber, peeled and thickly sliced
½ red onion, thinly sliced
½ cup crumbled feta cheese
¼ cup pitted kalamata olives
1 ½ teaspoons capers, rinsed
2 tablespoons red wine vinegar
1 very small clove garlic, minced
1 ½ teaspoons minced fresh dill
¼ teaspoon dried oregano
¼ teaspoon salt substitute
¼ teaspoon pepper
1 tablespoon olive oil

In a large bowl, toss the bell pepper, tomatoes, cucumber, onion, feta cheese, olives, and capers. In a small bowl, whisk together the vinegar, garlic, dill, oregano, salt substitute, and pepper. While whisking, slowly drizzle in the olive oil to make a thick dressing. Pour the dressing over the salad, toss, and serve immediately.

Tomato Salad

2 SERVINGS

3 medium tomatoes, quartered
½ medium green pepper, seeded and thinly sliced
½ medium onion, thinly sliced and separated into rings
¼ cup balsamic vinegar
½ teaspoon celery seed
½ teaspoon Dijon mustard
¼ teaspoon salt substitute
⅛ teaspoon pepper
1 large cucumber, peeled and sliced

In a large bowl, combine the tomatoes, green pepper, and onion. In a small saucepan, combine the vinegar, celery seed, mustard, salt substitute, and pepper; bring to a boil. Boil for 1 minute then pour over the vegetables. Let stand until mixture comes to room temperature. Stir in the cucumber. Cover and refrigerate for 2 hours or until chilled.

Asparagus Salad

2 SERVINGS

½ pound fresh asparagus, trimmed
2 cups mixed field greens
3 tablespoons balsamic vinegar
1 tablespoon fresh orange juice
1 tablespoon sesame seeds, toasted
1 teaspoon minced fresh ginger

Steam the asparagus until crisp-tender and immediately place asparagus in ice water. Drain and pat dry. Place salad greens on a serving platter; top with asparagus. In a small bowl, whisk the vinegar, orange juice, sesame seeds, and ginger. Drizzle over the salad.

Cucumber-Fennel Salad

2 SERVINGS

1 large cucumber, sliced
½ medium sweet onion, thinly sliced
1 small fennel bulb, thinly sliced
2 tablespoons fresh lemon juice
2 tablespoons olive oil
1 teaspoon chopped fresh dill
¼ teaspoon grated lemon zest
⅛ teaspoon pepper
⅛ teaspoon salt substitute

In a large bowl, combine the cucumber, onion, and fennel. In a jar with a tight-fitting lid, combine the lemon juice, olive oil, dill, lemon zest, pepper, and salt substitute; shake well. Pour over the cucumber mixture and toss to coat. Refrigerate until chilled.

Mediterranean Mint Salad

2 SERVINGS

3 tablespoons chopped fresh mint (any variety)
2 small cucumbers, diced
4 Roma tomatoes, diced
1 small red onion, minced
2 cloves garlic, minced
¼ cup sliced pitted kalamata olives
½ cup crumbled feta cheese
2 tablespoons olive oil
¼ cup fresh lemon juice
⅛ teaspoon salt substitute
⅛ teaspoon pepper

Toss the mint, cucumbers, tomatoes, onion, garlic, olives, and feta cheese together in a large bowl. In a separate bowl, whisk the olive oil, lemon juice, salt substitute, and pepper. Combine with the salad and chill at least 3 hours.

Very Quick Black Bean Salad

2 SERVINGS

½ of a 15-ounce can black beans, drained and rinsed
2 cups cherry tomatoes or grape tomatoes, sliced in half
2 green onions (scallions), minced
1 clove garlic, minced
2 tablespoons balsamic vinegar
1 tablespoon red wine vinegar

Combine everything in a large bowl and mix gently.

Zesty Lima Bean and Tomato Salad

2 SERVINGS

2½ cups cooked lima beans, fresh or frozen
2 tablespoons minced onion
2 large Roma tomatoes, seeded and chopped
¼ cup cider vinegar
2 tablespoons coconut oil
1 clove garlic, minced
1 teaspoon Dijon mustard
½ teaspoon dried crumbled sage
¼ teaspoon pepper

Combine the lima beans, onion, and tomatoes in a large bowl. In a small bowl, combine the vinegar, oil, garlic, mustard, sage, and pepper, and whisk to make the dressing. Combine the dressing and the salad. Allow to sit at least an hour before serving.

Recipe modified from original, courtesy of www.recipezaar.com.

Spinach-Chicken Salad

2 SERVINGS

2 medium tomatoes, cut in chunks
3 cups fresh spinach leaves
8 ounces grilled or baked boneless, skinless chicken breast, cut into
   1-inch cubes
1 tablespoon olive oil
1 tablespoon balsamic vinegar
⅛ teaspoon salt substitute

In a large bowl, toss the tomatoes with the spinach. Add the chicken, olive oil, vinegar, and salt substitute; toss.

Turkey Waldorf Salad

2 SERVINGS

8 ounces cooked turkey breast, cut into 1-inch strips
1 cup chopped red apple (about 1 apple)
1 cup sliced celery
1 cup red seedless grapes, halved
½ cup coarsely chopped walnuts
⅓ cup reduced-fat mayonnaise
¼ teaspoon salt substitute
¼ teaspoon pepper
4 cups mixed field greens
2 tablespoons chopped fresh parsley

In a large bowl, combine the turkey, apple, celery, grapes, walnuts, and mayonnaise. Season with salt substitute and pepper. Serve on a bed of greens. Sprinkle with chopped parsley.

VEGETABLE SIDE DISHES

When cooking vegetables, it is very important that you do not over-cook them. Overcooking will not only result in the loss of important nutrients, it will also alter the flavor. Light steaming, baking, and quick stir-frying are the best ways to cook vegetables. Do not boil vegetables unless you are making soup. In soup, many of the nutrients from the vegetables remain in the broth.

If fresh vegetables are not available, frozen vegetables are preferred over their canned counterparts. We prefer our vegetable side dishes fairly simple—steamed yams, carrots, broccoli, asparagus, potatoes, and other vegetables are just great on their own. Nonetheless, we are providing some additional favorite vegetable recipes here for your enjoyment.

Oven-Roasted Vegetables

2 SERVINGS

1 medium zucchini
1 medium summer squash
1 medium red bell pepper
1 medium yellow bell pepper
1 pound fresh asparagus, trimmed
1 medium red onion
3 tablespoons olive oil
1 teaspoon salt substitute
¼ teaspoon pepper

Preheat the oven to 450°F. Cut the zucchini, summer squash, red bell pepper, yellow bell pepper, and asparagus into bite-sized pieces. Put the vegetables in a large baking dish, and toss with olive oil, salt substitute, and pepper. Spread in a single layer. Roast for 30 minutes, stirring occasionally, until vegetables are lightly browned and tender.

Recipe modified from original, courtesy of www.recipezaar.com.

Lemon-Infused Green Beans

2 SERVINGS

1 pound fresh green beans, trimmed
1 red onion, cut into thin wedges
2 cloves garlic, thinly sliced
2 tablespoons olive oil
3 tablespoons fresh lemon juice
1 teaspoon salt substitute
¼ teaspoon pepper

In a partially covered microwave-safe dish, microwave the green beans and 1 tablespoon water for 4 minutes on high. In a skillet over medium heat, cook the onions and garlic in the olive oil for 3 minutes or until lightly browned. Add the green beans and 2 tablespoons of the lemon juice and cook until tender, stirring occasionally. Stir in the salt substitute and pepper. Sprinkle with the remaining tablespoon lemon juice.

Cherry Tomato and Zucchini Sauté

2 SERVINGS

1 tablespoon olive oil
3 small zucchini, halved lengthwise and thinly sliced
2 cups cherry tomatoes, halved
2 green onions (scallions), sliced
2 teaspoons balsamic vinegar
¼ teaspoon salt substitute
⅛ teaspoon pepper
2 tablespoons chopped fresh basil

Heat the olive oil in a large nonstick skillet over high heat. Add the zucchini and cook, stirring, for 1 minute. Add the tomatoes, green onions, and balsamic vinegar. Cook, stirring, for 1 to 2 minutes or until zucchini is crisp-tender and tomatoes are heated through. Season with salt substitute and pepper. Sprinkle with basil and serve immediately.

Recipe modified from original, courtesy of www.recipezaar.com.

Roasted Broccoli with Lemon and Garlic

2 SERVINGS

1 pound broccoli florets
2 tablespoons olive oil
2 tablespoons fresh lemon juice
¼ teaspoon salt substitute
⅛ teaspoon pepper
1 teaspoon minced garlic
½ teaspoon grated lemon zest

Preheat the oven to 500°F. In a large bowl, toss the broccoli with 1 tablespoon of the olive oil, 1 tablespoon of the lemon juice, the salt substitute, and pepper. Arrange the florets in a single layer in a baking dish and roast, turning once, for 12 minutes or until just tender. Meanwhile, in a small saucepan, heat the remaining olive oil, add the garlic and lemon zest. Cook, stirring, for about 1 minute. Let cool slightly and stir in the remaining lemon juice. Place the broccoli in a large bowl, pour the lemon dressing over it, and toss to coat.

Recipe modified from original, courtesy of www.recipezaar.com.

Asparagus with Thyme

2 SERVINGS

1 clove garlic, halved
1 ½ pounds asparagus spears, trimmed
1 tablespoon olive oil
¼ teaspoon dried thyme
¼ teaspoon salt substitute
¼ teaspoon pepper

Preheat oven to 400°F. Rub the cut sides of the garlic over the inside of a 13 by 9-inch baking dish, then place the garlic in the dish. Add asparagus to the dish and drizzle with the olive oil. Sprinkle the asparagus with thyme, salt substitute, and pepper. Toss gently and roast for 20 minutes, stirring once.

Shredded Zucchini

2 SERVINGS

4 or 5 zucchini
1 ½ tablespoons olive oil
3 or 4 cloves garlic, minced
2 teaspoons chopped fresh dill
2 tablespoons crumbled feta cheese
¼ teaspoon salt substitute
¼ teaspoon pepper

Shred the zucchini on the coarsest side of a grater. Heat the olive oil in large skillet, then add the zucchini and garlic. Sauté on medium heat, tossing often for about 5 minutes or until the excess moisture has evaporated. The zucchini should be bright green and firm-tender. Add the dill, feta, salt substitute, and pepper. Serve immediately.

WHOLE GRAIN RECIPES

Perhaps the healthiest manner in which to enjoy the nutritional benefits of whole grains is simply by boiling or steaming them with the help of a double-boiler or grain steamer. However, the most common method is to bring the appropriate amount of water to boil in a pot with a fitted lid, add the whole grain, bring to a boil again, reduce the heat, cover, and simmer for the prescribed amount of time (see "Guide to Cooking Whole Grains").

Whole grains are great diet foods because they are low in calories, high in fiber, and high in complex carbohydrates. But the key once again is portion control. You must keep the amount of whole grains consumed at any meal to less than one cup. Since cooking whole grains in water results in a tremendous increase in their water content, they are quite satiating due to their high bulk. Whole grains can be used as breakfast cereals, side dishes, casseroles, or as part of the main entree.

GUIDE TO COOKING WHOLE GRAINS

Grain (1 cup dry)	Cups Liquid*	Cooking Time (minutes)	Yield
Amaranth seeds	2½	20 to 25	2½ cups
Barley, flakes	2	30 to 40	2½ cups
Barley, hulled	3	75	3½ cups
Barley, pearl	3	50 to 60	3½ cups
Buckwheat	2	15	2½ cups
Cornmeal (fine grind)	4 to 4½	8 to 10	2½ cups
Cornmeal (polenta, coarse, grits)	4 to 4½	20 to 25	2½ cups
Millet, hulled	3 to 4	20 to 25	3½ cups
Oat bran†	2½	5	2 cups
Oat groats†	3	40 to 50	3½ cups
Oat, rolled	2	15	2½ cups
Oat, steel-cut	2	30	2½ cups
Quinoa†	2	15 to 20	2¾ cups
Rice, brown basmati	2½	35 to 40	3 cups
Rice, brown, long grain	2½	45 to 55	3 cups
Rice, brown, quick	1¼	10	2 cups
Rice, brown, short grain	2 to 2½	45 to 55	3 cups
Rice, wild	3	50 to 60	4 cups
Rye, berries or cracked grain	3 to 4	60	3 cups
Rye, flakes	2	10 to 15	3 cups
Spelt, kernels	3	60	2½ cups
Sorghum	2½	45 to 55	3 cups
Triticale, whole berries	3	105	2½ cups
Triticale, rolled (flakes) or cracked	2	15	2½ cups
Wheat, bulgur	2	15	2½ cups
Wheat, couscous (instant)	1	5	2 cups
Wheat, cracked	2	20 to 25	2¼ cups
Wheat, whole berries	3	120	2½ cups

* Use boiling water, juice, or broth
† Add to *cold* water, bring to boil, and simmer.

Barley Risotto

4 SERVINGS

2 cloves garlic, minced
½ onion, chopped
1 tablespoon olive oil
1 cup sliced mushrooms
1½ cups pearl barley
¼ cup white wine
4 cups vegetable stock
1 cup diced fresh tomatoes
Salt substitute and pepper
1 cup peas (shelled fresh or thawed frozen)
½ cup grated Romano cheese

Sauté the garlic and onion in the olive oil until softened. Add the mushrooms and cook until browned. Add the barley and cook for 5 minutes, stirring occasionally, until lightly toasted. Add the wine, 3 cups of the stock, the tomatoes, and salt substitute and pepper to taste. Bring to a boil, cover, and simmer 25 minutes, stirring occasionally. If using fresh peas, add the peas and some additional broth if all the liquid has been absorbed and simmer an additional 10 to 15 minutes; if using frozen peas, check for dryness, add stock if necessary, and simmer 10 to 15 minutes. Add the thawed peas and stir well. Stir in the cheese, and more salt substitute and pepper if needed. Serve immediately.

Comfort Food Rice

4 SERVINGS

1 teaspoon olive oil
1 cup brown rice
¼ cup chopped green onions (scallions)
½ cup chopped cilantro
1 clove garlic, minced
1 teaspoon salt substitute
1 teaspoon cayenne pepper or ½ hot chile pepper, seeded and minced
2½ cups water, vegetable broth, or chicken broth

Add the olive oil to a medium saucepan placed over medium heat and warm for 1 minute. Add the rice and sauté, stirring almost constantly, until the rice begins to turn clear and just a little brown on the edges. Add the green onions, cilantro, garlic, salt substitute and cayenne and sauté for 1 minute. Add the water, stir, and cover tightly. Reduce the heat to medium-low and cook for 40 minutes. Lift the lid and check to ensure the rice is thoroughly cooked. If not, re-cover, turn the heat to very low and let the pan sit on the warm burner for a few minutes. Remove from the heat and fluff with a fork when the rice is tender.

Flavorful Oat Burgers

12 SERVINGS

4 cups water
½ cup reduced-sodium soy sauce or tamari
½ cup nutritional yeast
1 large onion, diced small
1½ teaspoons garlic powder
1 tablespoon dried oregano
1 tablespoon dried basil
4½ cups old-fashioned oats
½ cup coarsely ground pecans
Olive oil cooking spray

Preheat the oven to 350°F. Bring the water, soy sauce, yeast, onion, garlic powder, oregano, and basil to a boil in a large saucepan. Reduce the heat to low and stir in the oats and nuts. Cook for about 5 minutes, until the water is absorbed. Let cool.

Coat a 13 x 9-inch nonstick baking pan with olive oil spray, then spread the mixture. Bake evenly in the pan for 25 minutes. Use a non-scratch utensil to cut the mixture into 12 burgers. Flip them over. Bake for 20 minutes more. Serve in whole-grain buns with all the fixings (low-fat versions, of course). Extras can be frozen.

Fantastic Brown Rice

8 SERVINGS

3 cups brown rice
2 eggs, lightly beaten
6 cups water
1 tablespoon olive oil

Preheat the oven to 350°F. Combine the rice and eggs in a large non-stick skillet and sauté stirring constantly over medium heat, until the mixture is dry. Add the water and oil and bring to a boil. Pour into deep, large baking dish. Bake uncovered for 30 minutes, cover with foil, and bake 30 minutes more. Do not stir or disturb.

Moroccan Barley

6 SERVINGS

1 ⅓ cups pearl barley
4 cups water
1 teaspoon salt substitute
1 tablespoon olive oil
1 cup sliced onions
½ cup sliced celery
2 cloves garlic, minced
2 carrots, sliced
1 medium zucchini, sliced
1 medium green bell pepper, seeded and cut into squares
1 cup broccoli florets
One 15½ ounce can chickpeas, drained
2 cups vegetable broth
2 teaspoons reduced-sodium soy sauce
2 teaspoons fresh lemon juice
½ teaspoon ground coriander
¼ teaspoon ground ginger
⅛ teaspoon cayenne pepper
2 tablespoons cornstarch, dissolved in 3 tablespoons water
Chopped cilantro, for garnish (optional)

To cook the barley, place the barley, water, and salt substitute in a large saucepan. Bring to a boil. Cover and cook on low heat for 45 minutes, or until the barley is tender and the liquid is absorbed. Set aside to keep warm.

To cook the vegetables, heat the oil in large, heavy saucepan over medium heat. Add the onions, celery, and garlic and sauté 3 to 4 minutes. Add the carrots, zucchini, green pepper, broccoli, chickpeas, broth, soy sauce, lemon juice, coriander, ginger, and cayenne. Bring to boil. Cover and simmer 10 to 15 minutes, or until the vegetables are tender. Stir in the cornstarch mixture and cook, stirring, until thickened. Spoon the barley around the edge of a deep platter. Pour the vegetables into the center. Garnish with cilantro, if desired, and serve.

Terrific Tuna Pasta Salad

4 SERVINGS

One 8-ounce package whole-wheat or brown-rice pasta shells
One (10-ounce) package frozen peas
2 green onions (scallions), minced
2 tablespoons low-fat mayonnaise
¾ cup plain nonfat yogurt
1 tablespoon Dijon mustard
1 clove garlic, minced
Salt substitute and pepper
1 (6-ounce) can tuna in water, drained

Cook the pasta according to package directions. Drain and set aside. In a small saucepan, cook the peas according to package directions. Drain and set aside. In a large bowl, combine the green onions, mayonnaise, yogurt, mustard, garlic, and salt substitute and pepper to taste. Mix lightly. Add the tuna, pasta, and peas and toss all the ingredients together. Cover and refrigerate until serving time.

Mexican Barley and Hominy

12 SERVINGS

2 teaspoons olive oil
1 cup chopped onions
4 fresh Anaheim chiles, seeded, deveined, and chopped
4 fresh jalapeño chiles, seeded, deveined, and chopped
8 cups chicken broth
1 cup pearl barley
One 29-ounce can hominy, drained and rinsed
Two 7-ounce containers salsa verde, or 1¾ cups of your favorite salsa
    verde recipe
½ teaspoon ground cumin
Shredded Cheddar cheese, for garnish (optional)
Finely chopped green onions (scallions), for garnish (optional)

In a large saucepan with a lid, heat the oil over medium heat. Sauté the onions and chiles for 5 minutes, stirring occasionally. Add 4 cups of the broth and the barley. Bring to a boil. Reduce the heat, cover, and simmer for 30 minutes. Stir in the remaining broth, the hominy, salsa, and cumin. Cook for 20 minutes longer. Ladle the soup into bowls and top with shredded cheese and green onions, if desired. Makes great leftovers.

LEGUME (BEAN) RECIPES

Legumes are often called "poor people's meat;" however, they might be better known as "healthy people's meat." Compared to grains, legumes supply about the same number of total calories, but usually provide two to four times as much protein. Many people shy away from legumes because they often cause increased intestinal flatulence (gas) or intestinal discomfort. The flatulence-causing compounds in legumes are primarily compounds known as oligosaccharides, which are composed of three to five sugar molecules linked together in such a way that the body cannot digest or absorb them. Because the body cannot absorb or digest these oligosaccharides, they pass into the intestines where bacteria break them down producing a gas by-product. Navy and lima beans are generally the most offensive, while chickpeas are the least because of their lower levels of oligosaccharides.

The amount of oligosaccharides in legumes and therefore the amount of flatulence produced by legumes can be dramatically reduced by proper cooking. See "Guide to Cooking Dried Beans," page 234, for guidance in properly cooking legumes. If, after following these instructions, you still experience increased flatulence when you eat legumes, you may wish to try a commercial enzyme preparation called Beano.

Although most legumes can be purchased precooked in cans, cooking your own offers significant economical as well as possible health benefits if the canned beans are full of sodium (salt). Cooking your own legumes will produce three times the amount on a cost basis compared to canned products.

Dried legumes, with the exception of lentils, are best prepared by first soaking them overnight in water to cover by at least one inch. This is best done in the refrigerator to prevent fermentation. Soaking will usually cut the cooking time dramatically. If soaking overnight is not possible, here is an alternate method: Place the beans in water in a saucepan, bring to a boil for at least 2 minutes, and then set aside to soak for at least 1 hour. Be forewarned, however, that beans cooked using the quick soak method may split or develop a slightly mushy consistency. For beans that retain an even shape, ideal texture, and tender, creamy bite without mushiness, overnight soaking is the optimal method. Beans that have not been presoaked may need some additional water, about one-quarter to one-half cup per cup of beans, to replace the water that evaporates as steam during their longer cooking process.

Before cooking presoaked beans, regardless of soaking method, skim off any skins that floated to the surface, drain the soaking liquid, and then rinse the beans with clean water. The beans should be brought to a gentle boil and then simmered with a minimum of stirring to keep them firm and unbroken. A pressure cooker or slow cooker can also be used for convenience. Regardless of cooking method, do not add any seasonings that are salty or acidic, such as vinegar, wine, tomatoes, or citrus fruits and their juices, until after the beans have been cooked since adding them earlier will make the beans tough and greatly increase the cooking time.

Whenever possible, use the cooking liquid as well as the beans in your recipes. Vitamins from the beans leach into the cooking water, resulting in significant loss of nutrients. For instance, about 35 percent of most of the B vitamins including 50 percent of the folic acid will leach into the liquid when beans are cooked for one hour and fifteen minutes.

If you are running short on time, you can always use canned beans in your recipes. If the beans have been packaged with salt or other additives, simply rinse them to remove these unnecessary additions. Canned beans need only to be heated briefly for hot recipes, while they can be used as is for salads or prepared cold dishes.

GUIDE TO COOKING DRIED BEANS

Beans (1 cup)	Cups Liquid*	Cooking Time (presoaked)	Cooking Time (unsoaked)	Yield
Adzuki (Aduki) beans	4	45 to 55 minutes	2 hours. If not done, add 20 to 30 minutes	3 cups
Anasazi beans	2½ to 3	45 to 55 minutes	1 hour	2¼ cups
Black beans	4	1 to 1½ hours	2 hours	2¼ cups
Cannellini (White kidney beans)	3	45 minutes	1 hour	2½ cups
Cranberry beans	3	40 to 45 minutes	1 hour	3 cups
Fava beans, skins removed	3	40 to 50 minutes	1 hour	1⅔ cups
Garbanzos (Chickpeas)	3 to 4	2 to 2½ hours	3 hours	2 cups
Great Northern beans	3½	1½ hours	2 hours	2⅔ cups
Peas, whole	6	1 to 2 hours	2 hours	2 cups
Kidney beans	3	1 hour	2 hours	2¼ cups
Lentils, brown	2¼	Not recommended	45 minutes to 1 hour	2¼ cups
Lentils, green	2	15 to 20 minutes	30 to 45 minutes	2 cups
Lentils, red	3	Not recommended	20 to 30 minutes	2 to 2½ cups
Lima beans, Christmas	4	1 hour	2 hours	2 cups
Lima beans, large	4	45 minutes to 1 hour	1½ to 2 hours	2 cups
Lima beans, small	4	50 to 60 minutes	1½ to 2 hours	3 cups
Peas, black-eyed	3	30 to 45 minutes	1 hour	2 cups
Peas, green split	4	45 minutes	1 hour	2 cups
Peas, yellow split	4	1 to 1½ hours	2 hours	2 cups
Mung beans	2½	1 hour	1½ hours	2 cups
Navy beans	3	45 to 60 minutes	1½ hours	2⅔ cups
Pink beans	3	50 to 60 minutes	1½ hours	2¾ cups
Pinto beans	3	1 to 1½ hours	2 hours	2⅔ cups
Soybeans	4	3 to 4 hours	1½ hours	3 cups

*Use water or broth

Chana Masala

3 SERVINGS

1 cup dried chickpeas or one 15-ounce can, drained and rinsed
2 tablespoons vegetable oil
½ teaspoon cumin seeds
½ teaspoon mustard seeds
1 teaspoon finely chopped fresh ginger
1 teaspoon finely chopped garlic
1 large onion, finely chopped
3 to 4 pinches asafetida powder (find at health food or Indian food stores)
½ teaspoon ground coriander
1 teaspoon red chili powder
½ teaspoon garam masala
¼ teaspoon ground turmeric
1 large tomato, chopped
2 tablespoons tamarind concentrate
1 tablespoon ghee or clarified butter
¼ teaspoon ground cinnamon
¼ teaspoon ground cloves
3 green chiles, chopped
1 tablespoon chopped cilantro, plus extra for garnish
1 small onion, sliced into thin rings, for garnish

If using dried chickpeas, soak overnight and cook until soft (2 to 3 hours). Heat the oil in a large, heavy skillet. Add the cumin and mustard seeds. Allow to crackle and sputter. Add the ginger, garlic, chopped onions, and asafetida. Fry until the onions are lightly browned. Add the coriander, chili powder, garam masala, and turmeric. Stir well. Add the tomatoes and cook until the oil separates. Add the drained chickpeas and stir well. Add the tamarind concentrate. Mix and cook until fairly dry. Set aside to keep warm. In a small saucepan, heat the ghee and add the cinnamon, cloves, and chopped chiles. Allow to pop a bit, then add to the skillet containing the chickpeas. Add 1 tablespoon chopped cilantro. Stir gently until well mixed. Garnish with more cilantro and the onion rings. Serve hot with brown rice or whole-wheat pita.

Sweet Potato–Black Bean Chili

6 SERVINGS

1 tablespoon olive oil
1 medium onion, chopped
½ pound lean ground turkey or chicken
2 cloves garlic, smashed
2 cups small cubes sweet potato (2 small or 1 large)
2 teaspoons ground coriander
2 teaspoons ground cumin
1 teaspoon dried oregano
½ teaspoon salt substitute
1 pinch ground cinnamon
Two 14.5-ounce cans diced tomatoes, undrained
1 jalapeño pepper, minced
Water or tomato juice, as needed
1 cup chopped red bell peppers
One 15-ounce can black beans, drained and rinsed
1 cup canned kidney beans, drained and rinsed
1 small zucchini, diced (about ¾ cup)
Fresh lime juice

Heat the olive oil in a large skillet or saucepan on medium-high heat. Add the onions, turkey, garlic, and sweet potatoes and cook for 5 minutes, stirring frequently. Add the coriander, cumin, oregano, salt substitute, and cinnamon, and sauté for another 5 minutes. Add the tomatoes and jalapeño and bring to boil. Reduce the heat to medium-low and simmer for 10 minutes. (You might need to add water or tomato juice if too much liquid evaporates.) Stir in the red peppers and simmer for 5 minutes. Add the black and kidney beans and simmer for an additional 5 minutes. Add the zucchini and cook for 5 minutes more. Stir in lime juice to taste.

Moroccan Chickpeas and Sweet Potatoes

4 SERVINGS

1 large onion, sliced thinly
3 cloves garlic, minced
1 tablespoon minced fresh ginger

2 tablespoon dry red wine or sherry

1 teaspoon ground cumin

1 teaspoon ground cinnamon

1 teaspoon paprika

½ teaspoon crushed red pepper flakes, or to taste

1 cup water or chickpea cooking liquid

½ teaspoon salt substitute

2 medium sweet potatoes (1 ½ pounds), peeled and cut into bite-size pieces

¼ cup diced dried apricots

2 cups cooked or canned chickpeas, drained

¼ cup raisins

2 tablespoons fresh lemon juice

¼ cup sliced almonds, toasted in a dry skillet

In a medium saucepan, combine the onions, garlic, ginger, and wine. Cover and sweat over low heat for 5 minutes. Add the cumin, cinnamon, paprika, and red pepper flakes and cook, uncovered, 1 minute longer. Add the water, salt substitute, sweet potatoes, and apricots. Bring to a boil, cover, and simmer until the sweet potatoes are just tender, about 15 minutes. Add the chickpeas, raisins, and lemon juice. Cook, stirring occasionally, for about 5 minutes, until the chickpeas are hot. Add the sliced almonds.

Roasted Vegetable Chili

8 SERVINGS

2 red bell peppers

3 cups frozen corn, thawed and drained

2 sweet potatoes, peeled and sliced ¼-inch thick

2 to 3 tablespoons olive oil

2 cloves garlic, minced

Two 28-ounce cans diced tomatoes

One 15-ounce can black beans, drained and rinsed

1 tablespoon ground cumin

1 teaspoon cayenne pepper, or to taste

1 tablespoon ground coriander

Preheat the broiler. Put the red peppers on a cookie sheet and place as close to the heating element as possible. Allow the skin to blister and turn completely black, turning the peppers as needed. (This step can also be done by putting the peppers on the grill or holding them over a gas burner set to high.) Once the skins are completely blackened, put the peppers in a bowl and cover with plastic wrap, or put them into a paper bag and fold the top over several times. Allow to cool for 10 minutes. Peel off the skin with your fingers. Cut off the tops and stems and empty out the seeds. Dice the peppers and set aside.

Spread the corn in a single layer on a cookie sheet lined with foil. Place under the broiler for a minute or two, rotating if necessary, until most of the corn has turned golden. Remove the cookie sheet, turn the kernels, and put back under the broiler for another minute. Set the corn aside.

Line the cookie sheet with clean foil. Place the sweet potato slices on the cookie sheet in a single layer. Put under the broiler for about 1 minute (you may want to rotate the cookie sheet after 30 seconds if one section is cooking much faster than the rest). Once the slices have become brown but not black, remove the cookie sheet, flip the slices, and replace under the broiler until brown. Set aside.

Add the olive oil to a large saucepan over medium heat. Add the garlic and cook for 1 minute. Reduce the heat and add the tomatoes, beans, peppers, corn, sweet potatoes, cumin, cayenne, and coriander. Simmer until the sweet potatoes are tender. If desired, serve topped with low-fat grated Cheddar cheese, low-fat sour cream, plain nonfat yogurt, chopped cilantro, or whatever you like.

Mediterranean Kalamata Hummus

4 SERVINGS

1 ½ cups canned chickpeas, drained and rinsed
¼ cup tahini (sesame seed butter)
2 cloves garlic
¼ cup fresh lemon juice
1 teaspoon cayenne pepper
4 tablespoons olive oil
¾ cup pitted kalamata olives

2 tablespoons capers, drained and rinsed
1 small red bell pepper, seeded and sliced
1 teaspoon ground cumin
3 tablespoons chopped fresh parsley

Combine the chickpeas, tahini, garlic, lemon juice, ¾ teaspoon of the cayenne, 2 tablespoons of the olive oil, the olives, capers, red pepper, ¾ teaspoon of the cumin, and 2 tablespoons of the parsley in a food processor and puree. Add enough cold water to achieve a spreadable consistency. Spoon the puree onto a shallow plate and smooth the top with a spoon. Drizzle with the remaining olive oil and strew with the remaining parsley. Sprinkle the remaining cumin and cayenne in a star pattern and serve with warm pita or veggies.

Black Bean Hummus

4 SERVINGS

One (15-ounce) can black beans, drained (reserve liquid)
2 cloves garlic, minced
¼ teaspoon salt substitute, or to taste
1 teaspoon ground cumin
¼ cup tahini
¼ cup fresh lemon or lime juice
1 tablespoon minced fresh parsley

Place the beans, garlic, salt substitute, cumin, tahini, and lemon juice in a blender or food processor and blend until smooth. Add a small amount of the reserved bean liquid for the desired texture, if necessary. Place in a serving dish and sprinkle with the parsley. Serve with pita bread, crusty bread, baked tortilla chips, or whole-grain crackers such as Wasa Crispbread.

Black Bean–Chicken Chili

8 SERVINGS

2 boneless, skinless chicken breast halves, cut into 1-inch pieces
1 cup chopped onions
1 cup chopped green bell pepper

2 cloves garlic, minced
2 tablespoons chicken broth
Four 14.5-ounce cans stewed tomatoes
Two 15-ounce cans black beans, drained and rinsed
1 teaspoon salt substitute
½ teaspoon hot sauce, or to taste
2 cups medium salsa
2 tablespoons chili powder
1 teaspoon ground cumin
Shredded low-fat Cheddar cheese, for garnish (optional)
Nonfat plain yogurt, for garnish (optional)

Simmer the chicken, onions, green peppers, and garlic in the 2 tablespoons of broth in a covered saucepan until the chicken is cooked through, 10 to 15 minutes. Add the tomatoes, black beans, salt substitute, hot sauce, salsa, chili powder, and cumin; mix well and simmer 30 to 45 minutes. Garnish with shredded low-fat cheese or plain yogurt, if desired.

Addictive Mexican Stew

5 SERVINGS

1 cup diced onions
1 or 2 cloves garlic, finely chopped
1 tablespoon olive oil
3 cups diced or shredded cooked skinless chicken or turkey
One 1.25-ounce package taco seasoning mix
Two 14½-ounce cans diced tomatoes, undrained
One 15-ounce can black beans or kidney beans, drained
One 8¾-ounce can whole kernel corn, drained
One 4-ounce can diced green chiles, drained
1 cup chicken broth
1½ teaspoons cornstarch

Cook the onions and garlic in the oil in large saucepan until tender. Add the chicken, taco seasoning, tomatoes, beans, corn, and chiles. Blend the broth and cornstarch; add to the saucepan. Bring to a boil; reduce the heat and simmer 15 minutes, stirring occasionally. Serve with whole-wheat tortillas or Wasa Crispbread.

Slow-Cooker Mediterranean-Style Beans and Vegetables

6 SERVINGS

One 15-ounce can great northern beans, drained and rinsed
One 15-ounce can red beans, drained and rinsed
5 teaspoons minced garlic
1 large onion, chopped
1 cup thinly sliced carrots
½ cup thinly sliced celery
2 cups diced fresh green beans
2 red chile peppers, chopped (remove as many or as few seeds depending
    on how much heat you want)
2 bay leaves
Salt substitute and pepper, to taste

Put everything in a large slow cooker and cook on low for 8 hours, or until the beans and vegetables are as soft as you like. (If you don't have a slow cooker, combine in a Dutch oven, cover, and bake at 175°F for 8 hours). Remove the bay leaves before serving.

Savory Chickpea Pancake (*Socca*)

2 SERVINGS

1 cup chickpea flour
½ teaspoon pepper
½ teaspoon salt substitute
1½ teaspoons minced, fresh rosemary leaves
1 cup warm water
3 tablespoons olive oil
½ medium onion, sliced

Place a heavy (preferably cast-iron) skillet in the oven and preheat to 450°F. In a large bowl, sift together the chickpea flour, pepper, and salt substitute. Add the rosemary. Whisk in warm water and 2 tablespoons of the olive oil. Cover the bowl and allow the batter to sit for at least 30 minutes. The batter should have the consistency of thick cream. Stir the onion into the batter. Remove the skillet from the oven. Add the remaining olive oil to the hot pan, pour the batter into the pan and bake for 12 to 15 minutes, or until the pancake is firm and the edges are set (the top may not be browned). Set the socca a few inches below your broiler for 1 to 2 minutes, just long enough to brown it in spots. Cut into wedges and serve hot with low-fat toppings of your choice.

Spicy Black Bean and Lentil Burgers

8 SERVINGS

1 cup dried black beans, or one 15-ounce can, drained and rinsed
1 cup dried lentils, or one 15-ounce can, drained and rinsed
½ small onion, chopped fine
3 cloves garlic, chopped fine
2 jalapeño peppers, seeded and minced
2 teaspoons chili powder
2 teaspoons salt substitute
1 teaspoon pepper
2 eggs, beaten
½ cup fine dry breadcrumbs
Cooking oil spray

If using dried beans and/or lentils, prepare them according to Guide to Cooking Dried Beans on page 234 and drain. Mash the beans and lentils well in large bowl. Stir in the onions, garlic, jalapeños, chili powder, salt substitute, pepper, eggs, and breadcrumbs. Roll the mixture into 8 patties. Spray a large, heavy skillet with cooking spray and heat over medium-high heat. Gently place the patties in the skillet and cook until firm and browned on the bottom. Carefully flip the patties and cook on the other side (5 to 8 minutes per side).

DINNER ENTREE RECIPES

The following dinner recipes take advantage of the principles of the Hunger Free Forever program to provide main courses that are very nutritious and filling. Remember, we want you also to include a salad or soup and a side vegetable with your meal.

Grilled Horseradish and Soy Salmon

2 SERVINGS

1 tablespoon low-sodium soy sauce
2 teaspoons prepared horseradish
Two 6-ounce salmon fillets, skin on

Mix the soy sauce and horseradish and spread over the salmon. Cover and refrigerate for 1 to 2 hours. Heat the grill to medium. Coat a fish basket or foil with cooking oil spray. Place the fillets in the basket or on the foil, skin side down. Grill for 6 to 8 minutes or until opaque in the center.

Thai-Style Tilapia

2 SERVINGS

¼ cup light coconut milk
3 whole almonds
½ small white onion, chopped
½ teaspoon ground ginger
⅛ teaspoon ground turmeric
½ teaspoon chopped fresh lemongrass, ¼ teaspoon dried, or ½ teaspoon grated lemon zest
⅛ teaspoon salt substitute
Two 4-ounce tilapia fillets
⅛ teaspoon black pepper
¼ teaspoon crushed red pepper flakes

In a food processor or blender, combine the coconut milk, almonds, onion, ginger, turmeric, lemongrass, and ⅛ teaspoon salt substitute. Process until smooth. Heat a large nonstick skillet over medium-high heat. Season the fish fillets with salt substitute and black pepper on both sides, then place them skin side up in the skillet. Pour the pureed sauce over the fish. Use a spatula to coat the fish evenly with the sauce. Sprinkle with the red pepper flakes. Reduce the heat to medium, cover, and simmer for about 15 minutes, until the puree is thickened and fish flakes easily with a fork.

Recipe modified from original, courtesy of www.recipezaar.com.

Fish with Veggies

2 SERVINGS

1 small zucchini, sliced
½ small onion, sliced
½ cup sliced mushrooms
2 lemon slices
1 tablespoon olive oil
⅛ teaspoon pepper
Large pinch garlic powder
Two 6-ounce fish fillets (red snapper, catfish, halibut, or cod)

Preheat the oven to 375°F. Sauté the zucchini, onion, mushrooms, and lemon slices in olive oil in a medium skillet until tender, about 3 minutes. Remove the lemon slices and set aside. Stir the pepper and garlic powder into vegetables. Spray a 13 by 9-inch baking dish with cooking oil spray. Place the fish in the baking dish and top with the vegetables and lemon slices. Bake until fish flakes easily, 30 to 35 minutes.

Grilled Chipotle-Lime Chicken Breasts

2 SERVINGS

¼ cup chipotle in adobo, minced
½ teaspoon adobo sauce from canned chipotles
2 tablespoons fresh lime juice
½ clove garlic, minced
1 tablespoon olive oil
⅛ teaspoon salt substitute
⅛ teaspoon pepper
1 pound boneless, skinless chicken breast halves (about 2)

Preheat a grill to medium-high. Mix the chipotle, adobo sauce, lime juice, garlic, olive oil, salt substitute, and pepper. Pour half into a resealable bag with the chicken and allow to marinate for 15 minutes. Set aside remaining marinade. Remove the chicken from the marinade (discard the marinade) and place on the grill. Grill the chicken 4 to 5 minutes, then flip over and cook another 4 to 5 minutes. Baste chicken with the remaining marinade. Immediately flip the chicken and drizzle on the other side. Grill until lightly browned, about 2 minutes. Remove from grill and pour any remaining marinade on top.

Recipe modified from original, courtesy of www.recipezaar.com.

Lemon Turkey Breasts

2 SERVINGS

1 tablespoon all-purpose flour
⅛ teaspoon salt substitute
⅛ teaspoon pepper
2 turkey breast cutlets pounded to ¼-inch thick (about ½ pound total)
1 tablespoon olive oil
1 tablespoon fresh lemon juice
1 tablespoon minced fresh parsley

Combine the flour, salt substitute, and pepper on a plate. Dip the turkey cutlets into the flour, coating evenly and shaking off the excess; set aside. Heat the olive oil in a large heavy nonstick skillet for 1 minute over medium-high heat. Add the cutlets and cook 1 to 2 minutes per side, until browned. Transfer to a plate lined with paper towels to drain. Reduce the heat to medium. Add the lemon juice and parsley to skillet, stirring with a wooden spoon to loosen the browned bits in the pan. Return the cutlets to skillet and cook 1 to 2 minutes, until heated through, basting often with the lemon-parsley sauce.

Turkey à l'Orange

2 SERVINGS

1 large orange, cut in half crosswise
¼ cup chicken broth
¾ teaspoon cornstarch
1 teaspoon olive oil
½ pound turkey breast cutlets, pounded to ½-inch thick
Salt substitute and pepper

Squeeze 2 tablespoons of juice from half of the orange. Cut the remaining orange into ¼-inch-thick slices and set aside. In a small bowl, combine the orange juice, broth, and cornstarch. Stir until blended, set aside. In a nonstick skillet, heat the oil over medium heat until hot. Add the turkey cutlets, sprinkle with salt substitute and pepper. Cook the cutlets for 5 to 8 minutes on each side, until lightly browned on the outside and no longer pink on the inside. Transfer to a platter and keep warm. Add the orange slices to the skillet and cook 2 minutes. Transfer the orange slices to the platter with the chicken. Stir the juice mix to blend. Add to the skillet. Heat to a boil for 1 minute, and add cutlets and orange slices back into the pan. Keep warm until ready to serve.

Bunless Chicken or Turkey Burgers

2 SERVINGS

½ pound extra lean ground chicken or turkey breast
2 tablespoons ketchup
2 tablespoons seasoned dry bread crumbs
1 tablespoon grated or finely chopped onion
1 egg white
1 clove garlic, minced
¼ teaspoon salt
¼ teaspoon pepper
Two ¼-inch slices red or yellow onion
Cooking oil spray

Preheat a grill to medium. In a large bowl, combining ground chicken, ketchup, bread crumbs, onion, egg white, garlic, salt substitute, and pepper. Mix well and shape into 2 patties about ½-inch thick. Coat the patties and onion slices with cooking oil spray. Grill the patties and onions for 6 to 7 minutes per side, until the patties are no longer pink in center.

Garlic-Lime Grilled Chicken with Mango Salsa

2 SERVINGS

2 boneless, skinless chicken breast halves
Juice of 1 large lime
2 cloves garlic, minced
½ tablespoon olive oil

SALSA
2 ripe mangoes, peeled, seeded, and chopped
2 very ripe Roma tomatoes, chopped
½ red or yellow bell pepper, seeded and chopped
½ serrano chile, seeded and minced (or to taste)
1 green onion (scallion), chopped
⅛ cup chopped cilantro
Juice of ½ lime
Pepper and salt substitute

2 cups steamed short-grain brown rice

Marinate the chicken with the lime juice, garlic, and olive oil in a resealable bag in the refrigerator for at least 2 hours or overnight. For the salsa, mix all the ingredients and set aside. Preheat a grill to low. Grill the chicken breasts, turning once, until no longer pink (discard the marinade). Place 1 cup rice on each plate. Cover with a chicken breast. Divide the salsa between the plates and serve.

ACKNOWLEDGMENTS

First of all, it is important for us to acknowledge all the researchers, physicians, and scientists who over the years have sought to better understand the complexity of diet and appetite control. In particular, we appreciate greatly the contribution of Dr. Vladimir Vuksan and his colleagues at the University of Toronto and St. Michael's Hospital.

Lastly, we are indebted to the team at Atria led by Judith Curr for believing in our vision and having the perseverance to make our book as reader-friendly and practical as possible. Thank you all!

MICHAEL T. MURRAY, N.D.   Most of all, I would like to acknowledge my wife, Gina. Her love, support, and patience are the major blessings in my life along with our wonderful children, Alexa, Zachary, and our littlest angel, Addison.

MICHAEL R. LYON, M.D.   To my dad, thanks for teaching me to believe that I can do great things with my life.

Appendix A: Trends in U.S. Food Consumption

During the twentieth century, food consumption patterns changed dramatically. Total dietary fat intake increased from 32 percent of calories in 1909 to 43 percent by the end of the century overall; carbohydrate intake dropped from 57 percent to 46 percent; while protein intake remained fairly stable at about 11 percent.

Compounding these detrimental changes are the individual food choices accounting for them. There were significant increases in the consumption of meat, fats, oils, sugars, and sweeteners in conjunction with the decreased consumption of noncitrus fruits, vegetables, and whole-grain products, but the biggest change in the last 100 years of human nutrition is the switch from a diet with a high level of complex carbohydrates, as found naturally occurring in grains and vegetables, to a tremendous and dramatic increase in the number of calories consumed from simple sugars. Currently, more than half of the carbohydrates being consumed are in the form of sugars such as sucrose (table sugar) and corn syrup, which are added to foods as sweetening agents. High consumption of refined sugars is linked to many chronic diseases, including obesity, diabetes, heart disease, and cancer.

TRENDS IN QUANTITIES OF FOODS CONSUMED PER CAPITA (POUNDS/YEAR)

Foods	1909	1967	1985	1999
Meat, poultry, and fish				
Beef	54	81	73	66
Pork	62	61	62	50
Poultry	18	46	70	68
Fish	12	15	19	15
Total	146	203	224	199
Eggs	37	40	32	32
Dairy products				
Whole milk	223	232	122	112
Low-fat milk	64	44	112	101
Cheese	5	15	26	30
Other	47	159	190	210
Total	339	450	450	453
Fats and oils				
Butter	18	6	5	5
Margarine	1	10	11	8
Shortening	8	16	23	22
Lard and tallow	12	5	4	6
Salad and cooking oil	2	16	25	29
Total	41	53	68	70
Fruits				
Citrus	17	60	72	79
Fresh	154	73	87	115
Processed	8	35	34	37
Total	179	168	193	231

(continued on next page)

TRENDS IN QUANTITIES OF FOODS CONSUMED
PER CAPITA (POUNDS/YEAR) *(continued)*

Foods	1909	1967	1985	1999
Vegetables				
Tomatoes	46	36	38	55
Dark green and yellow	34	25	31	39
Fresh	136	87	96	126
Processed	8	35	34	39
Total	**224**	**183**	**199**	**259**
Potatoes, white				
Fresh	182	67	55	49
Processed	0	19	28	91
Total	**182**	**86**	**83**	**140**
Dry beans, peas, nuts, and soybeans	16	16	18	22
Grain products				
Wheat products	216	116	122	150
Corn	56	15	17	28
Other grains	19	13	26	24
Total	**291**	**144**	**165**	**202**
Sugar and sweeteners				
Refined, sugar	77	100	63	68
Syrups and other sweeteners	14	22	90	91
Total	**91**	**122**	**153**	**159**

Appendix B: Glycemic Index, Carbohydrate Content, and Glycemic Load of Selected Foods

A complete list of the glycemic index (GI) and glycemic load (GL) of all tested foods is beyond the scope of this book—it would be a book in itself. So we have selected the most common foods. This listing will give you a general sense of what a high- and low-GL food is. The glycemic index for this listing uses glucose scored as 100.

We have listed the items by food groups, from low to high glycemic loads. You may notice that certain food groups are not included. For example, you won't see nuts, seeds, fish, poultry, and meats listed because individually, these foods have little impact on blood sugar levels due to their low carbohydrate content. In fact, these foods, particularly fats and oils, can lower the glycemic index of carbohydrate-rich foods by delaying absorption. (For more information on glycemic index and glycemic load, see page 51.)

If you would like to see an even more complete listing,

visit www.mendosa.com, a free Web site operated by medical writer David Mendosa. It is an excellent resource.

Food	Glycemic Load	Glycemic Index	Carbohydrates grams	Fiber grams
Beans (Legumes)				
Soybeans, cooked, ½ cup, 100g	1.6	14	12	7.0
Peas, green, fresh, frozen, boiled, ½ cup, 80g	2.0	48	5	2.0
White navy beans, boiled, ½ cup, 90g	4.2	38	11	6.0
Kidney beans, boiled, ½ cup, 90g	4.8	27	18	7.3
Peas, split, yellow, boiled, ½ cup, 90g	5.1	32	16	4.7
Lentils, ½ cup, 100g	5.3	28	19	3.7
Lima beans, baby, ½ cup cooked, 85g	5.4	32	17	4.5
Black beans, canned, ½ cup, 95g	5.7	45	15	7.0
Pinto beans, canned, ½ cup, 95g	5.8	45	13	6.7
Chickpeas, canned, drained, ½ cup, 95g	6.3	42	15	5.0
Kidney beans, canned and drained, ½ cup, 95g	6.7	52	13	7.3
Broad, frozen, boiled, ½ cup, 80g	7.1	79	9	6.0
Peas, dried, boiled, ½ cup, 70g	8.0	22	4	4.7
Baked beans, canned in tomato sauce, ½ cup, 120g	10.0	48	21	8.8
Black-eyed peas, soaked, boiled, ½ cup, 120g	10.0	42	24	5.0
Bread				
Multigrain, unsweetened, 1 slice, 30g	4.0	43	9	1.4
Oat bran & honey loaf, 1 slice, 40g	4.5	31	14	1.5
Sourdough, rye, 1 slice, 30g	6.0	48	12	0.4
Stoneground wholewheat, 1 slice, 30g	6.0	53	11	1.4
Wonder enriched white bread, 1 slice, 20g	7.0	73	10	0.4

Food	Glycemic Load	Glycemic Index	Carbohydrates grams	Fiber grams
Sourdough, wheat, 1 slice, 30g	7.5	54	14	0.4
Pumpernickel, 1 slice, 60g	8.6	41	21	0.5
Whole wheat, 1 slice, 35g	9.6	69	14	1.4
Healthy Choice Hearty 7-grain, 1 slice, 38g	10.0	56	18	1.4
White (wheat flour), 1 slice, 30g	10.5	70	15	0.4
Healthy Choice 100% whole grain, 1 slice, 38g	11.0	62	18	1.4
Gluten-free multigrain, 1 slice, 35g	12.0	79	15	1.8
French baguette, 30g	14.0	95	15	0.4
Hamburger bun, 1, 50g	15.0	61	24	0.5
Rye, 1 slice, 50g	15.0	65	23	0.4
Light rye, 1 slice, 50g	16.0	68	23	0.4
Dark rye, black, 1 slice, 50g	16.0	76	21	0.4
Croissant, 1, 50g	18.0	67	27	0.2
Kaiser roll, 1 roll, 50g	18.0	73	25	0.4
Pita, 1, 65g	22.0	57	38	0.4
Bagel, 1, 70g	25.0	72	35	0.4
Breakfast Cereals				
Oat bran, raw, 1 tablespoon, 10g	4.0	55	7	1.0
Bran with psyllium, ⅓ cup, 30g	5.6	47	12	12.5
Bran, ⅓ cup, 30g	8.0	58	14	14.0
All-Bran, ½ cup, 45g	8.5	33	26	7.0
All-Bran, ½ cup, 40g	9.2	42	22	6.5
Oatmeal (cooked with water), 1 cup, 245g	10.0	42	24	1.6
Shredded wheat, ⅓ cup, 25g	12.0	67	18	1.2
Mini Wheats (whole wheat), 1 cup, 30g	12.0	58	21	4.4
All-Bran Fruit 'n Oats, ½ cup, 45g	13.0	39	33	6.0
Weeta-Bix, 2 biscuits, 30g	13.0	69	19	2.0
Cheerios, ½ cup, 30g	15.0	74	20	2.0
Frosties, ¾ cup, 30g	15.0	55	27	1.0

Food	Glycemic Load	Glycemic Index	Carbohydrates grams	Fiber grams
Breakfast Cereals (*cont.*)				
Corn bran, ½ cup, 30g	15.0	75	20	1.0
Honey Smacks, ¾ cup, 30g	15.0	56	27	1.0
Wheatbites, 1 cup, 30g	16.0	72	22	2.0
Total, ¾ cup, 30g	16.7	76	22	2.0
Mini Wheats (blackcurrant), 1 cup, 30g	17.0	71	24	2.0
Puffed wheat, 1 cup, 30g	17.6	80	22	2.0
Bran flakes, ¾ cup, 30g	18.0	74	24	2.0
Kellogg's Crunchy Nut Cornflakes, 1 cup, 30g	18.0	72	25	2.0
Froot Loops, 1 cup, 30g	18.0	69	27	1.0
Cocoa Pops, ¾ cup, 30g	20.0	77	26	1.0
Team, 1 cup, 30g	20.5	82	25	1.0
Corn Chex, 1 cup, 30g	20.75	83	25	1.0
Just Right, ¾ cup, 30g	21.6	60	36	2.0
Corn flakes, 1 cup, 30g	21.8	84	26	0.3
Rice Krispies, 1 cup, 30g	22.0	82	27	0.3
Rice Chex, 1 cup, 30g	22.0	89	25	1.0
Crispix, 1 cup, 30g	22.6	87	26	1.0
Just Right Just Grains, 1 cup, 45g	23.5	62	38	2.0
Oat 'n Honey Bake, 1 cup, 45g	24.0	77	31	2.0
Raisin bran, 1 cup, 45g	25.5	73	35	4.0
Grape Nuts, ½ cup, 58g	33.3	71	47	2.0
Cake				
Cake, angel food, 1 slice, 30g	11.5	67	17	<1
Cake, sponge cake, 1 slice, 60g	14.7	46	32	<1
Cake, cupcake, with icing and cream filling, 1 cake, 38g	19.0	73	26	<1
Cake, chocolate fudge, mix, (Betty Crocker), 1 slice cake, 73g cake + 33g frosting	20.5	38	54	<1
Cake, banana cake, 1 slice, 80g	21.6	47	46	<1

Food	Glycemic Load	Glycemic Index	Carbohydrates grams	Fiber grams
Cake, Pound Cake, 1 slice, 80g	22.6	54	42	<1
Cake, French vanilla, (Betty Crocker), 1 slice cake, 73g cake + 33g frosting	24.4	42	58	<1
Cake, Lamingtons, 1 slice, 50g	25.0	87	29	<1
Cake, flan, 1 slice, 80g	35.85	65	55	<1
Cake, scones, made from mix, 1 scone, 40g	83.0	92	90	<1
Crackers				
Crackers, Corn Thins, puffed corn cake, 2, 12g	7.8	87	9	<1
Crackers, Kavli, 4, 20g	9.2	71	13	3.0
Crackers, Breton wheat crackers, 6, 25g	9.4	67	14	2.0
Crackers, Ryvita or Wasa, 2, 20g	11.0	69	16	3.0
Crackers, Stoned Wheat Thins, 5, 25g	11.4	67	17	1.0
Crackers, premium soda crackers, 3, 25g	12.5	74	17	0
Crackers, water crackers, 5, 25g	14.0	78	18	0
Crackers, graham, 1, 30g	16.0	74	22	1.4
Crackers, rice cake, 2, 25g	17.0	82	21	0.4
Fruit				
Cherries, 20 cherries, 80g	2.2	22	10	2.4
Plums, 3 or 4 small, 100g	2.7	39	7	2.2
Peach, fresh, 1 large, 110g	3.0	42	7	1.9
Apricots, fresh, 3 medium, 100g	4.0	57	7	1.9
Apricots, dried, 5–6 pieces, 30g	4.0	31	13	2.2
Kiwi, 1 raw, peeled, 80g	4.0	52	8	2.4
Orange, 1 medium, 130g	4.4	44	10	2.6
Peaches, canned, natural juice, ½ cup, 125g	4.5	38	12	1.5
Pears, canned in pear juice, ½ cup, 125g	5.5	43	13	1.5
Watermelon, 1 cup, 150g	5.7	72	8	1.0
Pineapple, fresh, 2 slices, 125g	6.6	66	10	2.8

Food	Glycemic Load	Glycemic Index	Carbohydrates grams	Fiber grams
Fruit (*cont.*)				
Apple, 1 medium, 150g	6.8	38	18	3.5
Grapes, green, 1 cup, 100g	6.9	46	15	2.4
Apple, dried, 30g	6.9	29	24	3.0
Prunes, pitted, 6 prunes, 40g	7.25	29	25	3.0
Pear, fresh, 1 medium, 150g	8.0	38	21	3.1
Fruit cocktail, canned in natural juice, ½ cup, 125g	8.25	55	15	1.5
Apricots, canned, light syrup, ½ cup, 125g	8.3	64	13	1.5
Peaches, canned, light syrup, ½ cup, 125g	9.4	52	18	1.5
Mango, 1 small, 150g	10.4	55	19	2.0
Figs, dried, tenderized (water added), 50g	13.4	61	22	3.0
Golden raisins, ¼ cup, 40g	16.8	56	30	3.1
Banana, raw, 1 medium, 150g	17.6	55	32	2.4
Raisins, ¼ cup, 40g	18.0	64	28	3.1
Dates, dried, 5, 40g	27.8	103	27	3.0
Grains				
Rice bran, extruded, 1 tablespoon, 10g	0.57	19	3	1.0
Barley, pearled, boiled, ½ cup, 80g	4.25	25	17	6.0
Millet, cooked, ½ cup, 120g	8.52	71	12	1.0
Bulgur, cooked, ⅔ cup, 120g	10.6	48	22	3.5
Brown rice, steamed, 1 cup, 150g	16.0	50	32	1.0
Couscous, cooked, ⅔ cup, 120g	18.0	65	28	1.0
Rice, white, boiled, 1 cup, 150g	26.0	72	36	0.2
Rice, Arborio risotto rice, white, boiled, 100g	29.0	69	35	0.2
Rice, basmati, white, boiled, 1 cup, 180g	29.0	58	50	0.2
Buckwheat, cooked, ½ cup, 80g	30.0	54	57	3.5
Rice, instant, cooked, 1 cup, 180g	33.0	87	38	0.2

Food	Glycemic Load	Glycemic Index	Carbohydrates grams	Fiber grams
Tapioca (steamed), 1 cup, 100g	38.0	70	54	<1
Tapioca (boiled with milk), 1 cup, 265g	41.0	81	51	<1
Rice, jasmine, white, long grain, steamed, 1 cup, 180g	42.5	109	39	0.2
Ice Cream				
Ice cream, low-fat French vanilla, 2 scoops, 50g	5.7	38	15	0
Ice cream, full-fat, 2 scoops, 50g	6.1	61	10	0
Jam				
Jam, no sugar, 1 tablespoon, 25g	6.0	55	11	<1
Jam, sweetened 1 tablespoon, 25g	8.0	48	17	<1
Milk, Soy Milk, and Juices				
Milk, full-fat, 1 cup, 250ml	3.0	27	12	0
Soy milk, 1 cup, 250ml	3.7	31	12	0
Milk, skim, 1 cup, 250ml	4.0	32	13	0
Grapefruit juice, unsweetened, 1 cup, 250ml	7.7	48	16	1.0
Nesquik chocolate powder, 3 teaspoon in 250ml milk	7.7	55	14	0
Milk, chocolate flavored, lowfat, 1 cup, 250ml	7.8	34	23	0
Orange juice, 1 cup, 250ml	9.7	46	21	1.0
Gatorade, 1 cup, 250ml	11.7	78	15	0
Pineapple juice, unsweetened, canned, 250ml	12.4	46	27	1.0
Apple juice, unsweetened, 1 cup, 250ml	13.2	40	33	1.0
Cranberry juice cocktail, 240ml	23.0	68	34	0
Coca Cola, 12 oz, 375ml	25.2	63	40	0
Soft drinks, 12 oz, 375ml	34.7	68	51	0
Milk, sweetened condensed, ½ cup, 160g	55.0	61	90	0

Food	Glycemic Load	Glycemic Index	Carbohydrates grams	Fiber grams
Muffins and Pancakes				
Muffins, chocolate, butterscotch, 1 muffin, 50g	15.0	53	28	1.0
Muffins, apple, oat, and raisin, 1 muffin, 50g	15.0	54	28	1.0
Muffins, apricot, coconut, and honey, 1 muffin, 50g	16.0	60	27	1.5
Muffins, banana, oat, and honey, 1 muffin, 50g	18.0	65	28	1.5
Muffins, apple, 1 muffin, 80g	19.0	44	44	1.5
Muffins, bran, 1 muffin, 80g	20.0	60	34	2.5
Muffins, blueberry, 1 muffin, 80g	24.0	59	41	1.5
Pancake, buckwheat, 1 medium, 40g	30.0	102	30	2.0
Pancake, enriched wheat, 1 large, 80g	39.0	67	58	1.0
Pasta				
Pasta, tortellini, cheese, cooked, 1 cup, 180g	10.5	50	21	2.0
Pasta, ravioli, meat-filled, cooked, 1 cup, 220g	11.7	39	30	2.0
Pasta, vermicelli, cooked, 1 cup, 180g	15.7	35	45	2.0
Pasta, rice noodles, fresh, boiled, 1 cup, 176g	17.6	40	44	0.4
Pasta, spaghetti, wholemeal, cooked, 1 cup, 180g	17.75	37	48	3.5
Pasta, fettucini, cooked, 1 cup, 180g	18.2	32	57	2.0
Pasta, spaghetti, gluten-free in tomato sauce, 1 cup, 220g	18.5	68	27	2.0
Pasta, macaroni and cheese, packaged, cooked, 1 cup, 220 g	19.2	64	30	2.0
Pasta, star pastina, cooked, 1 cup, 180g	21.0	38	56	2.0
Pasta, spaghetti, white, cooked, 1 cup, 180g	23.0	41	56	2.0

Food	Glycemic Load	Glycemic Index	Carbohydrates grams	Fiber grams
Pasta, rice pasta, brown, cooked, 1 cup, 180g	52.0	92	57	2.0
Sugars				
Fructose, 2 teaspoons, 10g	2.3	23	10	0
Honey, ½ tablespoon, 10g	4.6	58	16	0
Lactose, 2 teaspoons, 10g	4.6	46	10	0
Sucrose, 2 teaspoons, 10g	6.5	65	10	0
Glucose, 2 teaspoons, 10g	10.2	102	10	0
Maltose, 2 teaspoons, 10g	10.5	105	10	0
Snacks				
Corn chips, Doritos original, 50g	13.9	42	33	<1
Snickers, 59 g	14.3	41	35	0
Tofu frozen dessert (nondairy), 100g	15.0	115	13	<1
Real Fruit bars, strawberry, 20g	15.3	90	17	<1
Twix cookie bar (caramel), 59g	16.2	44	37	<1
Pretzels, 50g	18.3	83	22	<1
Mars bar, 60g	26.6	65	41	0
Skittles, 62g	38.5	70	55	0
Soups				
Tomato, canned, prepared, 1 cup, 220 ml	6.0	38	15	1.5
Black bean, 1 cup, 220ml	6.0	64	9	3.4
Lentil, canned, 1 cup, 220ml	6.0	44	14	3.0
Split pea, canned, prepared, 1 cup, 220ml	8.0	60	13	3.0
Vegetables				
Carrots, raw, ½ cup, 80g	1.0	16	6	1.5
Low glycemic vegetables	≈1.4	≈20	≈7	≈1.5
Asparagus, 1 cup cooked or raw				
Bell pepper, 1 cup cooked or raw				
Broccoli, 1 cup cooked or raw				
Brussels sprouts, 1 cup cooked or raw				
Cabbage, 1 cup cooked or raw				

Food	Glycemic Load	Glycemic Index	Carbohydrates grams	Fiber grams
Low glycemic vegetables (*cont.*)	≈1.4	≈20	≈7	≈1.5
Cauliflower, 1 cup cooked or raw				
Celery, 1 cup cooked or raw				
Cucumber, 1 cup				
Eggplant, 1 cup cooked				
Green beans, 1 cup cooked or raw				
Kale, 1 cup cooked, 2 cups raw				
Lettuce, 2 cups raw				
Mushrooms, 1 cup, cooked or raw				
Spinach, 1 cup cooked, 2 cups raw				
Tomatoes, 1 cup, cooked or raw				
Zucchini, 1 cup cooked or raw				
Carrots, peeled, boiled, ½ cup, 70g	1.5	49	3	1.5
Beets, canned, drained, 2–3 slices, 60g	3.0	64	5	1.0
Pumpkin, peeled, boiled, ½ cup, 85g	4.5	75	6	3.4
Parsnips, boiled, ½ cup, 75g	8.0	97	8	3.0
Corn on the cob, boiled, 1 medium, 80g	8.0	48	14	2.9
Corn, canned and drained, ½ cup, 80g	8.5	55	15	3.0
Sweet potato, peeled, boiled, 1 medium, 80g	8.6	54	16	3.4
Fresh corn kernels, ½ cup boiled, 80g	10.0	55	18	3.0
Potatoes, peeled, boiled, 1 medium, 120g	10.0	87	13	1.4
Potatoes, with skin, boiled, 1 medium, 120g	11.0	79	15	2.4
Yam, boiled, 1 medium, 80g	13.0	51	26	3.4
Potatoes, baked (no fat), 1 medium, 120g	14.0	93	15	2.4
Potatoes, mashed, ½ cup, 120g	14.0	91	16	1.0
Potatoes, instant mashed, prepared, ½ cup, 120g	15.0	83	18	1.0
Potatoes, new, unpeeled, boiled, 5 small, 175g	20.0	78	25	2.0
Cornmeal, cooked (polenta), ⅓ cup, 40g	20.0	68	30	2.0

Food	Glycemic Load	Glycemic Index	Carbohydrates grams	Fiber grams
Potatoes, french fries, fine cut, ½ cup, 120g	36.0	75	49	1.0
Gnocchi, cooked, 1 cup, 145g	48.0	68	71	1.0
Yogurt				
Yogurt, low-fat, artificial sweetener, 1 cup, 200g	2.0	14	12	0
Yogurt, with fruit, 1 cup, 200g	8.0	26	30	0
Yogurt, low-fat, 1 cup 200g	8.5	33	26	0

APPENDIX C: A QUICK GUIDE TO NON- AND LOW-CALORIE SWEETENERS

It is quite common for those with diabetes and those who want to lose weight to look to noncalorie and low-calorie sweeteners. While earlier versions of artificial sweeteners—saccharin and cyclamates (and later aspartame)—were embroiled in controversy over their safety, some of the newer products appear to be considerably safer. Certain natural sweeteners are even better choices. Here is a brief description of some of these alternative sweeteners, listed in order of our preference.

STEVIA

The most popular natural sweetener is stevia, which is extracted from the *Stevia rebaudiana* plant. Stevia contains a molecule known as stevioside that is 300 times sweeter than sugar and has an excellent safety profile.

Stevia products are used around the world for their incredible sweetening properties. However, since stevia has not been studied sufficiently in regard to safety to allow it to be categorized as generally recognized as safe (GRAS) by the U.S. Food and Drug Administration, it cannot be advertised as a sweetener in the United States. Instead, it is sold as a dietary supplement. Preliminary studies in animal models show that stevia can lower blood glucose levels and blood pressure, two effects of prime importance in dealing with diabetes.

Unfortunately, stevia does produce an aftertaste that some find unpleasant. There are several different brands of stevia, each with a slightly different taste. We recommend the SweetLeaf brand.

Fructose

You might be surprised that we are listing fructose as an acceptable sweetener. We want to be very clear here: We are referring specifically to pure crystalline fructose and not high fructose corn syrup. And we need to stress that we are referring to dosages of fructose less than 10 grams (about 2 teaspoons), and ingestion away from any other significant source of carbohydrates.

Fructose, or fruit sugar, is the primary carbohydrate in many fruits, maple syrup, and honey. In fact, the fructose content of most fruits and many vegetables is roughly 10 percent of their dry weight. Fructose is very sweet and is roughly 1.75 times sweeter than sucrose (white sugar). Although fructose has the same chemical formula as glucose $(C_6H_{12}O_6)$, its structure (shape) is quite different. In order to be utilized by the body, fructose must be converted to glucose within the liver.

Fructose is an acceptable sweetener at appropriate levels because it does not affect blood sugar control. The glycemic load calculation for 10 grams of fructose is only 2. In comparison, the glycemic load for a slice of bread is 10, an apple is 7, and a cup of rice is 26.

So you can see that 10 grams of fructose is not a problem even for people with diabetes or hypoglycemia. In fact, this low dosage is referred to as a catalytic amount of fructose. Studies conducted at Vanderbilt University and Tel Aviv University have shown that low-dose fructose significantly improves blood sugar control in both normal subjects and those with type 2 diabetes.

The reason that low dosages of fructose are so beneficial in improving glucose control is that it activates a key enzyme in the liver (glucokinase) that is the first step in the utilization of glucose. As a result of activation of this enzyme, a gradient is produced that basically pulls glucose into the liver cell from the bloodstream. Research has shown that the activity of this enzyme is reduced in type 2 diabetes. As a result, it leads to an increase in the production of endogenous glucose by the liver. Giving type 2 diabetics a catalytic amount of fructose significantly reduces glucose production by the liver and improves blood sugar control.

Fructose is also very effective in staving off the appetite. While studies have consistently shown that aspartame (NutraSweet, Equal), glucose, and sucrose actually increase appetite, fructose consumption has been shown to decrease the amount of calories and fat consumed. Typically, the studies will give the subjects food or drink containing an equivalent amount of fructose or other sweetener thirty minutes to two and a half hours before a meal and then allow them to consume as much food as they desire at a dinner buffet. The studies are designed in a double-blind fashion so that neither the observers nor participants know who has been given what. Consistently, subjects receiving the fructose-sweetened food or drink will eat substantially fewer calories and less fat compared to the groups receiving aspartame, sucrose, or glucose. This effect clearly indicates that fructose at appropriate levels can reduce appetite and make weight loss much easier to achieve.

POLYOLS

Sugar alcohols, or polyol sweeteners such as xylitol, erythritol, sorbitol, mannitol, and maltitol have become quite popular with the new focus on low-carb foods. These sweeteners are found in numerous food products, especially chocolate and sugar-free chewing gum, because they have a smooth mouthfeel and a sweet, cool, pleasant taste. They are also used in many sugar-free or "dietetic" candies, cake mixes, syrups, and other foods, and do not break down when heated.

In general, polyols are about 60 percent as sweet as sucrose, with one third fewer calories (2.6 calories per gram versus 4.0 for sugar). They do not cause cavities; in fact, xylitol actually prevents cavity formation. Because they are absorbed quite slowly and have a low glycemic index, polyols can be fantastic sweeteners for diabetics if low-glycemic food choices are used (see "The Glycemic Index of Polyols").

Polyol sweeteners are extremely safe at moderate dosages. However, because they are poorly absorbed at higher dosages (e.g., greater than 10 grams daily), they can cause gastrointestinal symptoms ranging from mild discomfort to severe diarrhea. Children, because of their smaller size, may be affected by even smaller amounts. Currently, the FDA requires a laxative notice only on the few products that may lead to the consumption of 50 grams or more of sorbitol daily, though some companies voluntarily label other products as well.

BE CAREFUL OF MISLEADING "NET CARBS" ON LABELS

The term "net carbs" refers to the total number of carbohydrates in a food minus fiber, glycerin, and sugar alcohols. In other words, it's the total number of carbs that can be absorbed and digested in the intestinal tract.

The general belief is that fiber, glycerin, and sugar alcohols don't raise blood glucose levels, but in reality, glycerin and some sugar alcohols can affect blood glucose. The problem with "net carbs" is that it implies a low glycemic index (GI), when in fact only two of the sugar alcohols, mannitol and erythritol, have a GI of zero. The GI of some of other polyols is quite high. For example, two maltitol syrups have a GI greater than 50, about the same as spaghetti.

The Glycemic Index of Polyols

Polyol	GI*	Calories/g
Maltitol syrup (intermediate)	53	3.0
Maltitol syrup (regular)	52	3.0
Maltitol syrup (high)	48	3.0
Polyglycitol (hydrogenated starch hydrolysate)	39	2.8
Maltitol syrup (high-polymer)	36	3.0
Maltitol	36	2.7
Xylitol	13	3.0
Isomalt	9	2.1
Sorbitol	9	2.5
Lactitol	6	2.0
Erythritol	0	0.2
Mannitol	0	1.5

* GI of glucose is 100.

XYLITOL

Of the polyols, xylitol deserves special mention. It is a sweetener that is approved for use in more than thirty-five countries including the United States. Our body manufactures up to 15 grams of xylitol each day, so xylitol is not a strange or artificial substance, but a normal part of everyday metabolism.

Xylitol occurs naturally in many fruits and vegetables and is most often commercially produced from birch trees. Pure xylitol is a white crystalline substance that looks and tastes like sugar. On food labels, it is classified broadly as a carbohydrate and more narrowly as a polyol or sugar alcohol. Like inulin and tagatose, xylitol is slowly absorbed and partially utilized. It provides roughly 2.4 calories per gram—40 percent less than sugar. It has a minimal effect on blood sugar and insulin levels, and has been shown to promote satiety and reduce caloric intake. More than twenty-five years of testing in widely different conditions confirms that xylitol use reduces tooth decay rates in both high-risk groups (high caries prevalence, poor nutrition, and poor oral hygiene) and low-risk groups (low caries incidence with all current prevention recommendations). It has no known toxicity, though it may cause cramping and loose stools in some individuals in dosages greater than 10 to 20 grams.

FRUCTOSE IN THE PRODUCTS WE HAVE DESIGNED FOR NATURAL FACTORS

Choosing an acceptable sweetener for the health-food market is a difficult proposition. Nobody wants to ingest unnecessary sweeteners or calories, but failure to use a sweetener makes a product considerably less appealing. The solutions are limited.

For example, while something as natural sounding as "rice syrup solids" may sound and look good on a label, it is really not an acceptable choice. The chief components of rice syrup solids are glucose and maltose. These sugars are immediately absorbed in the body. The glycemic load of these sugars is 10 (remember, fructose was 2), but because they are not as sweet as fructose, higher levels are usually required. It basically takes at least three times as much rice syrup solids to impart the same amount of sweetness as fructose—that results in fifteen times the glycemic load.

After weighing all available options, we have chosen to use fructose alone or in combination with stevia extract and/or xylitol as the sweetening agent in the powdered drink mixes we have designed for Natural Factors, including SlimStyles. The key point to remember is that issues with fructose relate entirely to dosage. Remember that because fructose is 1.75 times sweeter than sucrose, it requires significantly less to impart sweetness, especially when combined with xylitol and/or stevia. Low dosages of fructose actually enhance blood sugar control. In fact, the glycemic response to the SlimStyles Weight Loss Drink Mix has been assessed at the University of Toronto and the University of Sydney and was shown to have no effect on blood sugar levels (zero glycemic impact).

Luo Han Guo (*Momordica grosvenorii*)

The fruit extract from this plant native to southern China is nearly 300 times sweeter than sugar and has been used as a natural sweetener in China for nearly 1,000 years. The sweet taste of luo han guo comes mainly from compounds known as mogrosides. These compounds normally make up about 1 percent of the flesh of the fresh fruit. Through extraction, a powder containing 80 percent mogrosides can be obtained. This 80 percent extract is the form most widely available. Luo han guo is classed by the FDA as a GRAS (generally recognized as safe) product. There are no restrictions on consuming the fruit or its extracts. We give the recommended use level of moderate simply because the highly concentrated extract has only been available relatively recently and more time is needed to ensure that it can be safely consumed in greater quantities.

RANKING THE NONSUGAR SWEETENERS

Sweetener	Other Names	Recommended Use Level	Quick Comments
Stevia	SweetLeaf	Liberal	A natural sweetener extracted from the *Stevia rebaudiana* plant, it is 300 times sweeter than sucrose. Technically, stevia is a dietary supplement because it has not been evaluated or approved by the FDA as a sweetener. Preliminary studies show that stevia may have blood sugar–lowering and blood pressure–lowering effects. It does exert a mild to unpleasant aftertaste.
Fructose (pure, crystalline)		Moderate	The amount must be less that 10 grams (about 2 teaspoons) and away from other significant sources of carbohydrate
Xylitol and other polyols (maltitol, sorbitol, mannitol, erythritol)		Moderate	Polyols are roughly 60% as sweet as sucrose. They are poorly absorbed and do not break down when heated. Larger amounts—for example, a single intake of more than 10 to 30g, or a total daily intake of more than 40 to 80g—may produce a laxative effect.
Luo Han Guo		Moderate	The fruit extract from this plant native to southern China is nearly 300 times sweeter than sugar and has been used as a natural sweetener in China for nearly 1,000 years.
Sucralose	Splenda	Moderate	Sucralose is composed of sucrose with newly attached chlorine molecules. It is 600 times sweeter than sucrose and does not break down when heated.

Aspartame	NutraSweet, Equal	Conservative	A controversial sweetener that is reported to receive more complaints at the FDA than any other food substance. It is made from two amino acids naturally found in foods, phenylalanine and aspartic acid. Aspartame is 200 times sweeter than sucrose, but it loses sweetness when heated.
Acesulfame K	Sunett, Sweet One	Restrictive	Made from vinegar, acesulfame K is structurally similar to saccharin. It is 200 times sweeter than sucrose and is not broken down by the body.
Saccharin	Sweet 'n Low	Restrictive	Saccharin was initially removed from the market over fears that it was a carcinogen. It is 300 times sweeter than sucrose. Because of safety concerns, it is not recommended during pregnancy.

Appendix D: Frequently Asked Questions About PolyGlycopleX (PGX)

What Is PGX?

PolyGlycoplex (PGX) is a proprietary blend of three natural viscous, nonstarch polysaccharides that act synergistically to develop a higher level of viscosity greater than other dietary viscous fibers known. This blend forms a unique gel matrix that is maintained in the gastro-intestinal tract. Unlike many fiber-containing natural health products, PGX does not lose its gel-like viscosity in either acidic stomach or alkaline intestinal environments.

PGX is produced in a sophisticated process—induced viscosity technology via the EnviroSimplex method—in a conditioned chamber that collides the ingredients in an exact and precise proportion. The entire processing is pharmaceutical industry–based and strictly adheres to principles of good manufacturing practices (GMP). Every polysaccharide complex of PGX is an entity on its own and with its perfect composition and particle sizes contributes to maximum viscosity.

What Are the Physiological Benefits of PGX?

The physiological benefits exerted by PGX relate to its nature as a highly viscous nonstarch polysaccharide (fiber) with a very high water-

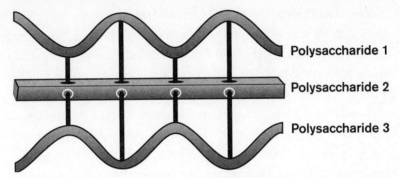

Figure D.1. The three polysaccharides of PGX bind together at side bonds to form an interlocking matrix. PGX is unique in that it represents proper blending and combining of the polysaccharides so that the side bond of the coils will link with the side bonds from the other polysaccharides coils, thereby working together to form a stable gel matrix with exceptionally high viscosity.

holding capacity. When consumed with food, PGX absorbs significant quantities of water, thus increasing the volume of gastric content and promoting an early sense of satiety even when food portions are decreased. PGX also increases food viscosity, thus slowing the rate at which food is digested and absorbed. This leads to beneficial effects such as prolongation of after-meal satiety and normalization of postprandial blood glucose and insulin excursions. This effect is in keeping with research demonstrating that the greater a fiber's viscosity, the more effective it will be in reducing the glycemic response to foods.[1]

In the colon, PGX is highly "prebiotic" in that it promotes growth of healthy bacteria and production of short-chain fatty acids (SCFA), substances that are vitally important to colon health.[2] The primary SCFA produced by bacterial action on PGX is propionate, which has been shown to increase production of bifidobacteria, suppress the growth of undesirable microbes such as *Candida albicans*, and lower stool pH. Propionate is also taken up by the liver and may help decrease production of cholesterol and free fatty acids. As a viscous polysaccharide, PGX also increases excretion of bile acids. With lower levels of bile in the bloodstream, additional bile acids are produced by the liver from blood cholesterol, lowering blood cholesterol levels.

WHY SHOULD I INCORPORATE PGX INTO MY DIET?

PGX is an excellent source of dietary fiber. In 2004, the average person in the United States and Canada consumed about 13 grams of dietary fiber per day.[3,4] The dietary reference intake of fiber for those 19 to 50 years old is 25 grams for women and 38 grams for men. Unfortunately, to achieve the greatest benefit, the additional dosage required (e.g., 20 grams or more) is often difficult to achieve with other fiber supplements. Moreover, it is difficult to obtain highly viscous fibers from our day-to-day food choices. In contrast, PGX is an easy and convenient way to add viscous soluble fiber to your diet, as it can be added to any meal or snack by mixing it into any beverage or sprinkling it onto moist food.

WHAT ARE THE CLINICALLY PROVEN HEALTH BENEFITS ASSOCIATED WITH PGX?

PGX and its prototype compositions have been studied for over fifteen years at the University of Toronto and Risk Factor Modification Centre at St. Michael's Hospital in Toronto, Canada, by Dr. Vladimir Vuksan and his research group. (Previous names used in Dr. Vuksan's publications include konjac-mannan, konjac-mannan polysaccharide mix, viscous fiber blend, and viscous polysaccharide blend.) This polysaccharide blend has now been further developed and refined into a commercially applicable product under the PGX logo. It is important to note that its mechanisms of action, properties, and health benefits remain, and continue to be supported with further laboratory research and clinical investigations. The Canadian Center for Functional Medicine has been using PGX extensively in various weight-loss programs and other medical interventions in regular medical and dietetic practice in order to investigate further its potency and the practicality of its application as learned from a clinical research setting.

Research surrounding the health effects of PGX has been done on healthy, overweight, and obese individuals, as well as people with type 2 diabetes and metabolic syndrome. Reported benefits include:

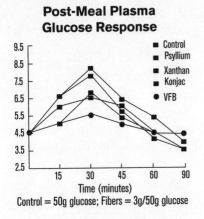

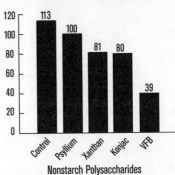

Figure D.2. Effects of adding 3g of different soluble nonstarch polysaccharides on postprandial glycemia when added to a 50g oral glucose load. Control is a 50g oral glucose load done alone.[8] Note: Viscous Fiber Blend (VFB) was the prototype for PGX.

- Reduced postprandial blood glucose levels (lowering the glycemic index of foods when consumed with PGX) and insulin concentrations[5,6,7]
- Increased insulin sensitivity and reduced body fat[8]
- Lower blood cholesterol levels[9,10]
- Reduced appetite and food intake[11]
- Healthy weight loss of 0.5 to 2 pounds per week[12]
- Reduced risk factors associated with metabolic syndrome[7,8]
- Improved bowel regularity

WHO SHOULD ADD PGX TO THEIR DIETS?

Against the backdrop of rising rates of obesity, metabolic syndrome, and type 2 diabetes, everyone would benefit from PGX, including those who want to:

- Reduce their risk of developing diabetes and/or cardiovascular disease
- Minimize their potential for metabolic syndrome or pre-diabetes
- Lower insulin resistance

- Better manage blood glucose levels, especially in type 2 diabetes
- Moderate high cholesterol levels, whether or not they are on cholesterol-lowering medication
- Achieve healthy weight loss (0.5 to 2 pounds per week)
- Cut food cravings and reduce their intake of extra calories

Dietary supplementation with PGX improves cardiovascular disease risk factors and reduces relative risk of cardiovascular disease in three population groups: healthy individuals and those with metabolic syndrome or type 2 diabetes. This conclusion is based on three studies that involved PGX, from which the relative risk for cardiovascular disease was calculated using the Framingham equation. Results showed that PGX reduced cardiovascular risk by 11 percent in type 2–diabetic subjects, by 21 percent in subjects with metabolic syndrome, and by 31 percent in healthy subjects.[9]

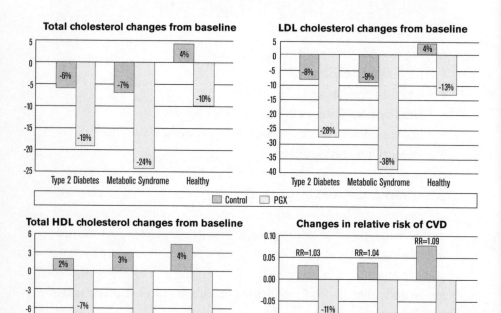

How Much PGX Should I Take Per Day?

To take full advantage of the health benefits associated with PGX, a recommended 2.5 to 5 grams should be taken with meals. Alternatively, 2.5 grams can be taken with healthy snacks or smaller meals throughout the day.

What Are the Common Side Effects of PGX?

When people first begin taking PGX, they may experience some gas, loose stools, transient diarrhea, abdominal bloating, or even some constipation. Others start on the full dose (10 to 15 grams per day) and experience no side effects, depending on the tolerability of their gut and microflora already existing in the colon. Overall, it can take the body and digestive tract from three to five days to adjust to the addition of higher quantities of PGX to the diet. To minimize side effects, 2.5 grams once or twice per day is recommended as a starting dose, which can be gradually increased to target levels. For those following a low-fiber diet, it is recommended they start on PGX slowly and increase the amount very gradually.

When enough water is consumed (between 8 and 12 ounces [375 and 500ml] per 5 grams), side effects are greatly minimized. It is important to drink a sufficient quantity of water with or immediately after each PGX serving.

Are There Any Contraindications with Common Medications?

PGX can slow the rate of absorption of foods and therefore it can theoretically do the same with medications. It is recommended that any oral medication be taken one hour before PGX and two to three hours after consuming the product. People with diabetes must monitor their blood sugar and may need to adjust medication accordingly, as PGX helps control blood sugar and may lessen the need for medications or insulin over time. It is recommended they consult a physician prior to adjusting their own medication. In some cases with those on medications for diabetes, with higher intakes of PGX blood glucose could drop below baseline and cause hypoglycemia.

If a person needs to take their medication in the morning with breakfast, they can take PGX with a midmorning snack, at lunch, and at dinner time. If a person is taking an array of medications, it may be appropriate to recommend that they consult with their physician prior to taking PGX.

Who Should Not Use PGX?

- Anyone who cannot compensate for a large intake of water, such as individuals with renal diseases and congestive heart failure
- Anyone on a large number of medications that need to be taken with food and/or without food, unless advised by physician
- Persons with gastrointestinal disorders who have difficulty swallowing, esophageal stenosis, or preexisting bowel abnormalities such as gastrointestinal strictures or impaired mobility, as they may be at risk for throat or esophageal blockage or bowel obstruction. Individuals with any gastrointestinal diseases or who have undergone gastrointestinal surgeries should consult their physician before taking PGX.
- Pregnant or lactating women should discuss PGX use with their healthcare professional.

Does Taking PGX Lower Mineral Bioavailability?

Research regarding the effects of PGX on mineral bioavailability is currently unavailable. Nonetheless, there is little or no evidence that PGX could cause mineral deficiency. Only in studies using insoluble dietary fibers have reductions in the bioavailability of some minerals been shown. In fact, some health experts have concluded that absorption is improved through the gastrointestinal tract with the consumption of high nonstarch polysaccharides or high-fiber diets. As supportive evidence to their conclusions the following points can be made:

1. Current evidence suggests that moderate fiber intake does not cause nutrient deficiencies, especially when consumed with a well-balanced diet.[4]
2. Research on glucomannan, one of the main ingredients of PGX, reports no reductions in mineral absorption.[13,14,15]
3. Phytic acid from cereal fibers or insoluble, nonviscous dietary fibers has been found to depress the absorption and retention of several minerals.[16] Since PGX does not contain phytic acids, it is

unlikely to affect mineral bioavailability. Fermentable fibers such as PGX have been shown to be nondigestible by human enzymes in the small intestine. In the large intestine they are fermented into short-chain fatty acids, which have been shown to increase mineral absorption.[17,18,19,20,21,22]

In summary, it would appear that dietary supplementation of PGX for extended periods does not adversely affect mineral balance.

How Is PGX an Improvement over Other Fiber Supplements/Products on the Market?

Some fibers on the market are nonthickening and thus offer none of the benefits associated with viscosity. Those that are viscous are less palatable since they develop viscosity and thicken very fast, making food and beverages unpleasant for consumption. Others have a bad taste, color, and/or grainy texture that make them less palatable. PGX is easy to use, natural, colorless, and has no distinctive odor or taste. Also, unlike some soluble fibers that thicken immediately upon contact with liquids, PGX granules develop viscosity at a much slower rate, so it is easy to mix into foods and beverages. This slower viscosity development reduces concerns of PGX expanding and obstructing the throat or esophagus because thickening likely occurs lower down in the gastrointestinal tract, such as in the stomach and small intestine.

Is PGX Simply a Weight-Loss Diet Product or Food Fad?

Definitely not. PGX is a volumetric and viscous fiber that can be easily incorporated into a wide number of eating patterns and lifestyles. PGX is easy to apply and can be used as a healthy supplement at home, on vacation, in a restaurant, or at a friend's for dinner. Eating a healthy balanced diet is always recommended, but for successful weight loss, many people need simple and practical help. Although there are many key considerations in a healthy weight-management program, including portion control and increased physical activity, PGX may assist with reductions in appetite, increased satiety, stabilization of blood glucose and cholesterol levels.[8,11]

References

1. D.J. Jenkins, et al, "Dietary Fibers, Fiber Analogues, and Glucose Tolerance: Importance of Viscosity," *British Medical Journal* (May 27, 1978): 1392–1394.

2. A.L. Jenkins, S. Panahi, A. Azatagagha, A. Rogovik, and V. Vuksan, "Effects of Different Fibers on Bowel Habits in Healthy Individuals," presented at FASEB (Federation of American Societies for Experimental Biology), Washington D.C., 2006.

3. Ministry of Industry, "Food Statistics 2005," *Statistics Canada Catalogue No. 21-020-XIE.* 5 (1), 2006.

4. United States Department of Health and Human Services and U.S. Department of Agriculture, *Dietary Guidelines for Americans 2005, 6th edition* (Washington D.C.: U.S. Government Printing Office, January 2005).

5. Glycemic Index Laboratories, "Determination of Glycemic Index Lowering Potential of PGX in Liquid and Solid Food Formulations," August 2, 2006.

6. A.L. Jenkins, L. Morgan, U. Zdravkovic, J. Sievenpiper, and V. Vuksan, "Importance of Administration Mode of Viscous Fiber (VF) on Postprandial Glycemia," presented at the 8th Annual Canadian Diabetes Association (CDA)/Canadian Society of Endocrinology and Metabolism (CSEM) Professional Conference, Quebec City, October 2004, poster #93.

7. V. Vuksan, et al, "Beneficial Effects of Viscous Dietary Fiber from Konjac-mannan in Subjects with the Insulin Resistance Syndrome: Results of a Controlled Metabolic Trial," *Diabetes Care* 23 (2000): 9–14.

8. V. Vuksan, M. Lyon, P. Breitman, and J. Sievenpiper, "3-Week Consumption of a Highly Viscous Dietary Fiber Blend Results in Improvements in Insulin Sensitivity and Reductions in Body Fat: Results of a Double Blind, Placebo Controlled Trial," presented at the 64th Annual Meeting of the American Diabetes Association, Orlando, Florida, June 4–8, 2004.

9. A. Rogovik, A.L. Jenkins, P. Breitman, and V. Vuksan, "A Blend of Highly Viscous Polysaccharides Decreases Relative CVD Risk in Three Population Groups," Natural Health Product Research Conference, Toronto, 2006.

10. V. Vuksan, et al, "Konjac-Mannan (Glucomannan) Improves Glycemia and Other Associated Risk Factors for Coronary Heart Disease in Type 2 Diabetes. A Randomized Controlled Metabolic Trial," *Diabetes Care* 22 (1999): 913–919.

11. P. Breitman, V. Vuksan, and M. Lyon, "Impact of Meal Replacement

Viscosity on Appetite and Ad-Libitum Food Consumption in Normal Weight Adolescents," presented at the 8th Annual Canadian Diabetes Association (CDA)/Canadian Society of Endocrinology and Metabolism (CSEM) Professional Conference, Quebec City, October 2004.

12. Canadian Center for Functional Medicine, PGX weight-loss program, unpublished results.

13. H. Yun-Hua, Z. Li-Shi, Z. Hong-Ming, W. Rui-Shu, and Z. Yin-Zhu, "Influences of Refined Konjac Meal on the Levels of Tissue Lipids and the Absorption of Four Minerals in Rats," *Biomedical and Environmental Science* 3 (1990): 306–314.

14. M.Y. Zhang, S.S. Peng, Y.Z. Zhang, and Z.H. Wu, "Long-Term Animal Feeding Trial of the Refined Konjac Meal. I. Effects of the Refined Konjac Meal on the Calcium and Phosphorous Metabolism and the Bone in Rats," *Biomedical Environmental Science* 8 (1995): 74–79.

15. C. Livieri, F. Novazi, and R. Lorini, "Usefulness of Highly Purified Glucomannan Fibers in Childhood Obesity, *La Pediatrica medica e chirurgica (Medical and Surgical Pediatrics)* 14 (1992): 195–198.

16. J.L. Greger, "Nondigestible Carbohydrates and Mineral Bioavailability," *Journal of Nutrition* 129 (1999): 1434S–1435S.

17. K.M. Behall, D.J. Scholdfield, K. Lee, A.S. Powell, and P.B. Moser, "Mineral Balance in Adult Men: Effects of Four Refined Fibers," *American Journal of Clinical Nutrition* 46 (1987): 307–314.

18. K.M. Behall, et al, "Effect of Guar Gum on Mineral Balances in NIDDM Adults," *Diabetes Care* 12 (1989): 357–364.

19. K.M. Behall, "Effects of Soluble Fibers on Plasma, Glucose Tolerance and Mineral Balance," *Advances in Experimental Medicine and Biology* 270 (1990): 7–16.

20. C. Coudray, et al, "Effects of Soluble or Partly Soluble Dietary Fibers Supplementation on Absorption and Balance of Calcium, Magnesium, Iron and Zinc in Healthy Young Men," *European Journal of Clinical Nutrition* 51 (1997): 375–380.

21. M. Tahari, et al, "Five-Week Intake of Short-Chain Fructo-Oligosaccharides Increases Intestinal Absorption and Status of Magnesium in Postmenopausal Women," *Journal of Bone and Mineral Research* 16 (2001): 2152–2160.

22. I.J. Griffin, P.M. Davila, and S.A. Abrams, "Non-Digestible Oligosaccharides and Calcium Absorption in Girls with Adequate Calcium Intakes," *British Journal of Nutrition* 87 (2002, Suppplement 2): S187–191.

APPENDIX E: WHAT TO LOOK FOR IN A MULTIPLE VITAMIN AND MINERAL SUPPLEMENT

While a health-promoting diet is an essential component of good health, so too is proper nutritional supplementation. While some experts say that you can theoretically meet all of your nutritional needs through diet alone, the reality is that most Americans do not come anywhere near the optimal levels. During recent years, the U.S. government has sponsored a number of comprehensive studies—HANES I, II, and III, Ten State Nutrition Survey, USDA nationwide food consumption studies, etc.—to determine the nutritional status of the population. These studies have revealed marginal nutrient deficiencies exist in a substantial portion of the U.S. population (approximately 50 percent) and that for some selected nutrients in certain age groups, more than 80 percent of the group consumed less than the Recommended Dietary Allowance (RDA).

These studies indicate the chances of consuming a diet meeting the RDA for all nutrients is extremely unlikely for most Americans. While it is theoretically possible that a healthy individual can get all the nutrition they need from foods, most Americans do not even come close to meeting all their nutritional needs through diet alone. In an effort to increase their intake of essential nutrients, many Americans look to vitamin and mineral supplements.

GIVING YOUR BODY THE TOOLS IT NEEDS

For optimum health, a high-quality multiple vitamin and mineral supplement is an absolute necessity. A high-quality supplement is one that provides optimal levels of both vitamins and minerals. Your body needs all of the important building blocks in order to build health. The following recommendations provide an optimum intake range to guide you in selecting a high-quality supplement. (Note that different vitamins and minerals are measured in different units. IU = International Units; mg = milligrams, mcg = micrograms.)

Vitamin	Range for Adults
Vitamin A (retinol)*	2,500–5,000 IU
Vitamin A (from beta-carotene)	5,000–25,000 IU
Vitamin B_1 (thiamin)	10–100mg
Vitamin B_2 (riboflavin)	10–50mg
Vitamin B_3 (niacin)	10–100mg
Vitamin B_5 (pantothenic acid)	25–100mg
Vitamin B_6 (pyridoxine)	25–100mg
Vitamin B_{12} (cobalamin)	100–400mcg
Vitamin C (ascorbic acid)	250–500mg
Vitamin D†	100–600 IU
Vitamin E (d-alpha tocopherol)	100–400 IU
Niacinamide	10–30mg
Biotin	100–600mcg
Folic acid	400–800mcg
Choline	10–100mg
Inositol	10–100mg

Mineral	Range for Adults
Calcium‡	250–1,000mg
Chromium	200–400mcg
Copper	1–2mg
Iodine	50–150mcg
Iron§	15–30mg
Magnesium	250–350mg

Mineral	Range for Adults
Manganese	1–5mg
Molybdenum	10–25mcg
Selenium	100–200mcg
Silica	1–5mg
Vanadium	50–100mcg
Zinc	15–20mg

* Women of childbearing age who may become pregnant should not take more than 2,500 IU of retinol daily due to the possible risk of birth defects. (Note: beta-carotene is safe during pregnancy and lactation.)
† People living in northern latitudes should supplement at the high range.
‡ Women should take 800 to 1,000mg of calcium to reduce the risk of osteoporosis.
§ Men and postmenopausal women rarely need supplemental iron.

To find a multiple vitamin and mineral formula that meets these criteria, read labels carefully. Be aware that you will not be able to find a formula that can provide all of these nutrients at these levels in one single pill—it would simply be too large. Usually it will require at least four tablets to meet these levels. While many "one-a-day" supplements provide good levels of vitamins, they are woefully insufficient in the levels of minerals.